OVERCOMING OSTEOARTHRITIS

MY HEALING JOURNEY

by

AUDREY G. BUCHANAN

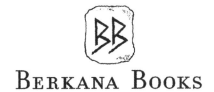

BERKANA BOOKS

Published by Berkana Books, PO Box 372,
Bowen Island, BC, V0N 1G0, Canada.

Cover design by Robert Grey.
Printed in Vancouver, BC, Canada by Benwell-Atkins Ltd.

Material from *The Artist's Way* by Julia Cameron,
copyright © 1992 by Julia Cameron, used by permission of
Jeremy P. Tarcher, a division of Penguin Putnam Inc.

Canadian Cataloguing in Publication Data

Buchanan, Audrey, 1927-
Overcoming osteoarthritis: my healing journey

Includes bibliographical references.
ISBN 1-894499-44-1

1. Osteoarthritis—Popular works. 2. Holistic medicine.
1. Title.

RC931-067B83 2000   616.7'223   C00-900707-5

DEDICATION

This book is dedicated to all my family and friends for their loving support and trust in my process, and to all those who are currently challenged by osteoarthritis.

A special thank-you to Olga Sheean, whose perceptive and sensitive editing skills brought this book to completion.

Thank you also to Batyah, who first suggested I tell my healing story, and to Dr Christine Bird, Carol Brophy, RMT, Dr David Bayley, Hélène Guenette, RMT, Réjèan Roy, Dr T. Wang, Evans Hermon, RN, Usha Thorne, and Dr John M. Davis, together with all those who gave of their gifts on my healing journey.

And lastly, but mostly, I wish to thank my son Russell, who patiently taught me to use the computer. His insightful support became a further shared, joyful experience.

Suddenly the bird whirled from its bough,
plunged headlong into space.
with a leap, my guide dived into the blue,
fell toward the flashing heavens, flew away.
Now the wave of fate had reached its peak,
now it tore away my heart,
now it broke in silence.
And already I was falling, I plunged, leaped,
I flew, wrapped in a cold vortex,
I shot, blissful and palpitating with ecstatic pain,
down through infinity to the mother's breast.

—Hermann Hesse

Contents

Preface

My journey to wellness took the form of physical, mental and spiritual healing methods—a holistic hologram for reversing illness and disease.

Holistic living is essentially the conscious act of taking responsibility for oneself, even to the point of recognizing that one has agreed to acquire a certain illness—perhaps unconsciously—in order to enhance self-awareness and knowledge through the healing process. When I first heard this theory, I thought it callous and lacking in compassion. However, I have since learned that the healing journey constitutes an invaluable process of discovery that involves delving into hitherto unexplored places and concepts in order to understand the deeper, and sometimes darker, side of one's nature.

By accepting the circles and spirals of growth, and then learning to love the myriad complex pieces that make up the God-self, one can know one's inner healing powers.

Telling my story uncovered me. Although I submitted my manuscript to several publishers in the hope of getting it published, I came to realize that my book was simply a continuation of my two decades' work as a Holistic Health Educator and Practitioner, which had been so rudely interrupted by osteoarthritis.

As the journey unfolded, I discovered that the interruption was but a prelude to a fuller, richer and healthier life than I could ever have imagined.

Note: Nothing in this book should be construed as advice for specific medical conditions, or as a substitute for medical care, where necessary.

Chapter 1 / My Life in Review

*Even as my fruits open, as my gifts become manifest, as I
mature in openness and love, I remember that I have
walked this path before, and will again.*
—Danny Pary, *the Essene Book of Days*

I was walking across my kitchen to the breakfast nook with a
pot of freshly made tea in my hand, when I began to feel the
hot pot slipping from my grasp. Like a slow-motion movie
scene, I watched the teapot smash to pieces, casting the hot,
wet tea leaves everywhere. I could still feel in my hands the
sense of the pot falling away from me and being helpless to
prevent it.

I mopped up the kitchen and left the house to go over
to the studio in the garden. I opened the door into my
beautiful workroom where I knew that I would not be
disturbed. The large octagonal window framed a Japanese-
like scene of descending pools fringed with planted rocks.
The young accolade cherry blossom trees were in full bloom,
and the stands of bamboo showed new green-tipped leaves.
This property had once housed a small derelict chicken farm
with various outbuildings. One of these had been converted
into the studio in which I now stood. In the stillness, I asked,
"What is happening to me?"

I settled into a comfortable chair, quieted my
breathing, and drifted into a reverie. Memories and images of
my past began to flow through me. I first saw myself as a
small, sturdy girl with healing hands, and recalled that this
was how the women of my mother's family referred to me.
My first real memory was of putting my hands on my

mother's head and neck when I knew she had a headache; after a while, I experienced the delicious sensation of the heaviness leaving her body. She would then smile at me with her bright blue eyes and say, "That's fine, that's fine," and I would go off about my business, giving the incident no further thought. When my father was partially blinded in an accident, my mother was required to go to work and I became the caretaker of my two younger brothers. There was a lot of work for me to do. My favourite getaway place was the local library. An avid reader, I would dip into the worlds that lay between the book covers as I walked home.

In my teen years, I became seriously ill due to an unknown bacterium, thought to have been brought to England by troops returning from the eastern war front. High temperatures and foul-smelling fevers left me completely debilitated with partial paralysis of my legs. The latest sulfa drugs were used to bring down the fevers, and my parents were advised that I was very seriously ill. At the crisis turning point, with a high temperature, I had a strange delirium-like experience, accompanied by a whooshing sensation in my chest. I felt myself being pulled up into a garden filled with light and had the distinct feeling that I was told I could not stay there. I was very disappointed about this, but did not mention the experience to anyone. Years later, I learned that I had had a near-death experience, and that the sensations I'd felt were quite normal, in such circumstances.

Lying listlessly on my bed in the garden, I remember hearing our family doctor telling my mother to be prepared for the possibility that I might not be able to walk again or live a normal life. But my mother replied confidently, "We shall start walking tomorrow," which we did! Each day, I walked slowly up the hill outside our house, counting the fence posts as I went, and then returned home to rest until the next day. This continued until my muscles became stronger. Several months after the illness, Dr Toop suggested that I be sent to his old Nanny and her husband for a period of convalescence. In the elderly couple's serene little home, with its lush garden, I was embraced by their deep compassion and the simple faith that permeated every small act as we moved through the days. There was much for me to absorb—books to read, herbs to learn about in the garden, and music to experience as Nanny Baker's husband played his violin in the evenings. Their warmth and generosity promoted a deep healing within me.

A few months later, I felt ready to put the illness behind me and to get on with my life. I asked our dear Dr Toop if I would pass the medical examination required if I were to apply to join Her Majesty's Forces. He replied that there were no visible signs of the illness, and that I appeared to have made a remarkable recovery. With just one look, he knew that this was my way of leaving home. In fact, I joined the Women's Auxiliary Air Force, where I met and later married Ross, my husband.

When I later returned to civilian life, I resumed my work as a private secretary. At the time I learned I was pregnant, I also discovered what for me was a life-changing book. It was about the joy of natural childbirth without the need for anaesthetics, written by Dr Grantley Dick Read. It included yoga-like postures and breathing techniques that I practised during my pregnancy. I remember telling my mother and two of her friends about the book over tea one day. They smiled indulgently at me, then exchanged meaningful glances with pursed lips, as if to say, "She will learn that it is not that easy." However, by good fortune, or Divine intervention, I discovered that, under the National Health plan, I was to be one of a small number of token patients to be allotted to a rather posh private nursing home. When the appointed birthing day arrived, and I had been settled in the labour room, I explained to the nurse on duty how I had prepared myself. I believe she assumed that I was a private patient and that arrangements had been made in advance for me to have a natural birth. Thus, after making me comfortable, she left me alone to work my way through the day. At eight minutes to six in the evening, Sister King came sailing through the door in her crisp white headdress, looking like a swan about to take flight. She announced briskly, "Well, my dear, you have done very well, but I have a special date at 6pm so I want you to give a good strong push to move things along." I did, and our lovely healthy son was born. It was the spring of 1951.

Barely a year later, we were on our way to Canada. My husband, a civil engineer, had accepted a post in Ontario. We gradually worked our way across the country from project to project until we reached Vancouver, British Columbia, where I eventually gave birth to a beautiful baby girl. Our little family was thriving.

These memories faded from my mind as I broke out of my reverie when I felt the need to move around. Wrapping a warm jacket around my shoulders, I went back outside, hugging myself, and made my way down the rhododendron path. When I came to my sitting log—my private place for contemplation—I sat and looked up into the Mother Tree, a tall cedar that had once been surrounded by the ever-encroaching bush. Another young tree had grown up around this one, looking as if it was clasping the older tree with its arms. With a little pruning, Ross had uncovered a beautiful natural sculpture. The two trees were wreathed in long shafts of sunlight that filtered through the surrounding trees, almost touching my feet, as if in a blessing. Because of the special magical quality of this place, we had decided to name it Thistledown.

Gradually, I became aware of the devas (nature spirits) all around me, and I cast my mind back to my first experience of their presence on this land. Ross and I were in the orchard, battling huge blackberry briars so long undisturbed that they had grown up through the fruit trees and back down to re-root themselves in the earth. As we hacked away at the colossal roots, Ross said in exasperation, "Can you think of an easier way to do this?" I replied, "I could ask the Blackberry Deva." "Good idea," Ross said, not entirely convinced it would help.

As a child, I had always been comfortable with the idea of nature spirits. (Many years later, my belief was confirmed when I heard Dorothy Maclean speak of her experiences with the deva kingdom in the Findhorn Gardens in Scotland.) So I took myself off to make contact with the Blackberry Deva. When I could feel her presence, I explained what we had come here to do with the land: we did not wish to harm it, but rather nurture it back to its natural beauty. I asked the deva if she would kindly arrange for the blackberry roots to surrender to us as we cleared the trees of their burden and, in return, we would set aside an area of the fruit garden where the blackberries could flourish undisturbed. Then Ross and I continued our clearing work and eventually removed all the deep roots with seemingly greater ease. We put our beehives next to the Deva's Patch, and this area always yielded the largest and juiciest blackberries at harvest time. I sent my gratitude to the devic kingdom each time I leaned into their blackberry bushes to pluck their proffered fruits.

A squirrel sitting above me chattered and threw down his empty fir-cone husks. I closed my eyes again and went back to the early 1960s—a time of awakening to an explosion of exciting ideas and information. Many people were expressing concern at the amount of pesticides being used in the earth which, in turn, were becoming absorbed by the plants grown in these soils, and ultimately ingested by the public at large. Research by Dr Adelle Davis had revealed an increasing number of unhealthy babies being born with a magnesium deficiency, which adversely affected their development. This valuable mineral became inert in the presence of chemical fertilizers and pesticides in the soil. Dr Davis also strongly advocated supplementing one's diet with vitamins and minerals.

Also at this time, I heard about the ancient Chinese healing art of acupuncture, which involved using needles to stimulate and balance the natural healing energy of the body. Then a neighbour gave me a book called *In Tune with the Infinite*, written by Ralph Waldo Trine. This inspiring discourse described a Universal spiritual path that encompassed diverse philosophies, without excluding any of them. As I became increasingly aware of the many different facets to human existence, I felt the need to learn more and to teach these principles to others. Within five years, I was teaching yoga and was also attending a wide variety of other courses and lectures. As a result, I was finally beginning to feel comfortable within myself, and with my surroundings and my community.

In the early 1970s, I was offered a job in an alternative school. Most of the pre-grad high school students there were bright, articulate, young people who had been 'turned off' by standard schooling. Our program re-framed the curriculum and we negotiated with students through self-responsible goal setting. It was a creative and rewarding time for everyone involved.

I moved on to study at the Holistic Health Institute in Santa Cruz, California, and began my real life's work in 1978, practising as a Holistic Health Educator and Practitioner the many forms of holistic healing of body/mind, spirit and soul.

In the summer of 1986, while walking with Ross in Vancouver's downtown Stanley Park, I injured my right wrist and thumb. We were walking in the rose gardens when the park sprinkler suddenly sprang to life. As we ran to avoid being drenched, we collided with each other. My right hand struck his chest, and my wrist hyper-flexed, overextending muscles and ligaments, and jolting the elbow, shoulder and neck up into the occiput (the two bones at the base of the skull). Within a couple of days, the discomfort seemed to have subsided and I continued with my work. Since much of my work involved Swedish Esalen massage and Shiatsu bodywork, my wrists and hands were important tools for me.

During the following year, I became increasingly aware of the pain in my wrists and thumbs, but I ignored it, not wanting to acknowledge that something more serious was developing. My work was going so well and was enthusiastically received by many in the community interested in holistic healing methods. So, too, were the healing gatherings we held at Thistledown. Many more people came to experience the healing work of people like Rev. Edward Oldring—the man who walked and talked with angels—and Gaston Saint-Pierre, who introduced us to the Metamorphic Technique (or Pre-natal Therapy), discovered by Robert St John, ND. (This method involved articulating a pattern within the spinal reflexes of the feet to release energies that were impeded during the gestation or pre-natal period; it provided yet another self-healing modality.)

Back in the present day, sitting on my log, I knew that my denial of what was happening to my hands was a normal initial reaction; the possibility of an incapacitating illness was not something I wanted to acknowledge. But now I knew it was time to move on.

I got up and stretched, feeling the growing chill in the air as the sun sank behind the trees. I was grateful for the quiet interlude I had given myself and for the sense of inner connectedness that had welled up in me. I took the path back to the house, past the pools where the darkening reflections on the water were shot with the silver-gold and orange movements of the languid koi fish.

It was time to face the truth, seek medical advice, and learn what I needed to know to meet this mounting challenge.

Chapter 2 / Finding Answers

The only thing that is required for a healing
is lack of fear.
—*A Course in Miracles*

My family physician ordered X-rays that showed a marked loss of connective tissue in both wrists and thumbs. His opinion was that I had osteoarthritis, a degenerative joint disease that indicates that the immune system is no longer functioning properly. It would only grow worse, with time. The body was unable to rebuild itself as fast as it was wearing down. I was given a prescription for painkillers.

Osteoarthritis is the most common type of arthritis and, with age, most people are likely to suffer from it to some degree.

There are at least two kinds of osteoarthritis: 'primary,' which develops without any triggering event, often affecting the hands, and occurring most commonly among women with a family history of arthritis; and 'secondary,' which develops after an injury or repeated strain or damage to a joint. Secondary osteoarthritis most often affects the larger joints, such as the knees, hips, and spine. It is not uncommon for someone to develop more than one type of arthritis.[1]

I realized I might never work with my hands in my profession again. I could not understand how, with my healthcare background, I could have acquired such an illness.

---

[1] *The Arthritis Handbook: the Complete Guide to Living a Healthy, Productive Life with Arthritis,* Theodor W. Rooney, D.O. & Patty Ryan Rooney.

I watched my diet, exercised regularly, did work I loved, and had a close community of supportive family and friends. Actually, I was somewhat embarrassed as well as angry that I had this condition. I saw myself as the one who gently massaged other people's arthritic limbs, and not as one who was incapacitated.

One of my biggest challenges was dealing with my frustration and anger. I had a huge fear of becoming helpless and dependent on others. I had to deal somehow with these emotions. In her book, *You Can Heal Your Life*, Louise Hay says that she considers feelings of frustration and anger to be one of the primary causes of osteoarthritis. When I first read this, I rejected the idea, but as I further explored the realm of emotions, I learned that uncovering deep-seated feelings do indeed have a great deal to do with the healing process of this—and any other—disease.

I stopped working. Many mornings I awoke with hands, wrists and elbows feeling hot, swollen, and stiff. If I over-exerted myself, a buzzing sensation could be felt anywhere in my body—from my toes to my jawbone. I became quickly fatigued and sad. The sadness was probably masking the anger that arose when I needed help to twist off jar lids, and when lifting heavy pots from the stove became increasingly difficult.

I decided to put together a daily program for myself, starting with a gentle massage using herbal oils. Once my limbs had softened and cooled from my touch, I started gentle stretching exercises, concentrating on my hands and wrists. Breathing exercises were followed by periods of deep relaxation. I began a diet of raw and steamed vegetables, avoiding the nightshade family of potatoes, peppers, eggplant and tomatoes. I continued eating fresh fruits and juices, and drank six-to-eight glasses of spring well water each day. I also stepped up my vitamin supplements. My joints gradually became cooler and less painful, and I made steady improvement.

In March of 1992, I was well enough to go with a friend on a tour of the Guatemalan Highlands and Costa Rica. Each morning on the journey, I rose early to do my stretching and breathing exercises. I visualized the forthcoming day, seeing myself dealing with each situation comfortably and joyfully. Then I sat in meditation for a few minutes, feeling focused and confident.

One evening, we were on our way to visit a coffee plantation high in the Costa Rican hills. As our bus travelled up a heavily potholed, winding hillside road, I saw a knapsack beginning to slide off the rack above our heads and stood up to grab it. Just at that moment, the bus went into a particularly deep pothole, causing me to hit my head and come down hard on my seat. Other than losing my breath for a moment, I felt fine. However, the seemingly minor incident was to have more serious implications later on.

Later in the journey, our group climbed up to the pyramids at Tikal, one of the main reasons I had come to Guatemala. In this lush, tropical setting, we hiked upwards for an hour or so, coming into a clearing where the pyramids soared skyward in all their dark, brooding splendour. It was a moving experience for me as I began to sense the archaic energies surrounding us.

As I walked around these towering structures, my mind was flooded with the sounds, smells, and images of some ancient gathering of people who seemed to be waiting for something to happen. I felt their fear and helpless anger. The energy then changed to the heavy numbness of surrender and the inevitability of ritual sacrifice.

I moved away, taking a path that led out of the temple enclosure, and groped in my bag for the rose quartz stone I carried there. With its familiar cool smoothness in my palm, I stepped off the path into the undergrowth and made a shallow hollow in the earth with the heel of my shoe. Kneeling down, I pressed my stone into the soil, asking that its heart-healing vibrations dissolve and heal the anguish of the former peoples of this land. As I stood up, I began to feel waves of peace spreading around me. I looked up into the trees and expressed my gratitude.

Back on the path, I breathed deeply and my chest felt wide open as I hurried to catch up to the group. Eating lunch, we were surrounded by the colours and sounds of nature, with brightly plumed birds flying above us in the trees, while below a dusty old anteater cadged titbits of food. We made our way back down the trail and were transported to a rest house where we were to stay for a couple of days.

Upon arrival, we were greeted by a bevy of toucans perched in the trees near our cabin. Grabbing my camera, I set off to take pictures of these exotic birds. However, in my haste, I slipped and fell. I slithered down a dry rocky bank, landing hard on my tailbone and the back of my head. My friend helped me to my feet and back to our cabin, where I asked her to prepare the homeopathic Rescue Remedy I carried with me for accident or shock.

The rest of our busy tour passed without incident. I had plenty of energy and none of the common intestinal problems suffered by some of our group. I attributed this in part to my morning regimen, vitamin supplements, and the ground flaxseed and lecithin granules with breakfast foods that I carried with me. I also carried Citricidal, an intestinal tract cleanser made from grapefruit seed. I used the liquid form to purify our drinking water and to wash the fruits and vegetables we bought in the local markets.

Shortly after I arrived home, I developed flu-like symptoms, aching joints and tiredness. One day, I suddenly felt an excruciating, blinding pain in my neck and right temple. I went to our family doctor and told him about the fall while away on holiday. He agreed to have X-rays taken. They clearly showed impaction of the second, third and fourth vertebrae and disc displacement in my neck. Once again, he prescribed pain-killers.

A month later, after Ross and I had returned from one of our Sunday walks, I went to work in the garden, only to find that I could not put weight on my right foot. My right hip and knee could not hold me up. Once again, I had X-rays taken and these showed more damage to my lower spine.

After five years of steady improvement since the diagnosis in 1987, it was hard to believe that a great deal more bone tissue had degenerated. It had probably been aggravated by my fall in Guatemala and the impact of the jolting bus. Now I was in constant discomfort and unable to walk far without a cane. I felt despondent about my physical progress, but I was also eagerly awaiting the birth of our first grandchild. Claire was born September 29, 1992, and when I held her in my arms for the first time, I resolved to learn everything I could to help me overcome this disease.

This was the real beginning of my healing journey. When I began writing this, Claire was nearly three years old—a beautiful, active and lively little girl. I hoisted up her little bottom to change diapers, I crawled into her play tent to read books with her, and I joined her in her first swim in the sea. I realized that the healing journey begins with the recognition and release of fear, anger, and sacrifice that harbour the seeds of our disease. Our healing is a many-faceted, many-coloured mosaic that resides within the wealth of our own unique experiences of the heart/mind. And as we explore these hidden realms within us, we find the way back to wholeness.

Chapter 3 / Attitudinal Shifts

The moment one definitely commits oneself,
then Providence moves too. All sorts of things occur to help
one that would otherwise never have occurred.
—Goethe

To shift old ways of thinking and behaviour requires changing one's perspective on life. The energy and focus for these changes usually comes from new or traumatic situations. As a species, we are resistant to change, but I needed to address my resistances as part of my commitment to the healing process.

There were four main attitudinal shifts that aided my recovery. They involved body, mind, spirit and emotions, and required making different choices, and letting go of that which no longer served me.

When I collided with Ross in Stanley Park, it became clear that, within my body, osteoarthritis was already eroding my bones. I denied the pain of this for a year in order to continue my work. X-rays produced a medical truth, but how I dealt with this trauma required more of me than taking drugs.

One of the first significant shifts in my attitude came through the study of *A Course in Miracles*. This book, based on Christian principles and the teachings of all the great masters, included 365 daily lessons, to be diligently studied and practised.

Several well-known authors, such as Ken Wapnick, Gerry Jampolsky, Dr Bernie Segal and Dr Deepak Chopra, to name a few, use the principles of this book to illustrate and support their theories on the nature of healing.

As children, many of us are taught that we must be 'good' and 'nice,' regardless of our feelings. We grow up with a distorted sense of what is right or good, in terms of our self-expression.

The *Course* offered me an opportunity to take responsibility for my own thinking, choose my own behaviour, and eventually recognize the value of our rich inner world.

We personally have a lot to do with how we experience or create our world. Thoughts and feelings that swirl around us in times of stress or crisis often create a sense of imbalance or vulnerability. Such feelings can provide us with useful information, especially when we have our own internal tools for re-framing the ways in which we respond to people and situations in life. Our inner dialogue helps us to view and practise life from a different perspective.

The most dynamic concept of the *Course*'s teachings is that there are only two emotions: love and fear—one being the opposite of the other. I am either scrunched up in fear (ie feeling rejected, sad or angry), or I am open and moving forward with life in a truthful, trusting and sharing way. But staying in this positive frame of mind is not easy. What do we do with the blame and judgements we carry from our past? That is what the daily lesson is for—to put into practice the desire not to carry the weight of these negative feelings and attitudes that hinder our well-being, happiness and creativity.

Behind the pain and suffering of illness is fear. If we can locate and understand the nature of our fear and release it, we have a better chance of moving into a place of love. But how and whom should we love? This is the hardest question of all for the answer is that we must love ourselves—contrary to our upbringing. Without this self-love, we cannot truly love others. Yet embracing love and acceptance of self and others brings countless rewards.

Another shift in attitude occurred with regard to my oil painting. I loved applying thick, juicy swaths of colour to a canvas as a means of expressing my inner feelings. When I found I could no longer hold a brush or use a palette knife properly, I was concerned that I would not be able to paint any more. But I wanted and needed to paint, so I considered using watercolours. Initially, I thought they would be difficult to master and that I would miss the tactile pleasure of oil painting. However, after learning some new techniques, I discovered the excitement of executing delicate washes of colour that I had never been able to achieve with oils. This new medium was magical!

After I stopped working and concentrated on my own healing process, Ross and I undertook another challenge— another attitudinal shift. We decided to give up our home, Thistledown, with its studios and large gardens, to make a quieter life for ourselves. After a week of house hunting and asking ourselves where we should go, an old childhood dream came back to me. I was about eight or nine years old and was standing alone on the beach saying goodbye on the last day of a family holiday by the sea. In my mind's eye, I could see and feel the hard ridges of sand beneath my feet and the transparent rings of water, touched with lacy foam, swirling around my ankles. I could hear myself saying out loud, "When I grow up and can do what I want, I will live by the seaside all the time, and never have to go home"—like all the lucky people who lived in that small seaside town.

On this day, many years later, after telling Ross about my dream, we began making enquiries into coastal properties. We were eventually led to a beachfront site at Roberts Creek, BC. The owners, we were told, had hitherto been adamant about not selling but, on the day we called, they were apparently having second thoughts. We made an offer that was accepted, and Ross and I designed a house for two with space for a studio we could share. We moved into the Seaside House in May 1988.

Letting go of emotional attachments to certain plans, or resurrecting old dreams seems to be part of the perpetual human dance of life. Although our path may seem random and sometimes chaotic, it rarely is. There is a grand universal design that unfolds effortlessly, once we surrender to it. And because nature abhors a vacuum, any emptiness we create should, ideally, be filled with new life patterns. I think it is the way we dance our destiny.

The daily physical practice of the *Course*'s teachings brings us to new levels of awareness and allows our perceptions to change, eventually creating whole new insights into our healing and co-creative abilities.

Chapter 4 / Detoxification

We must be willing to relinquish the life we've
planned, so as to have the life that is waiting for us.
—*Joseph Campbell*

When I was first diagnosed with osteoarthritis, my doctor prescribed an anti-inflammatory medication to reduce the burning sensation in the affected joints. It did bring some relief, but it also upset my stomach and made me feel very groggy, so I stopped taking it. Joint discomfort is often due to the accumulation of toxic wastes—as was the case with my thumbs, wrists and elbows.

One form of toxic waste is the residue left by poorly digested, refined, de-natured foods. Such foods are particularly unsuitable for some individuals, as are the chemical additives used in the processing of many food products. I learnt the hard way just how much stress and discomfort certain foods can cause for an arthritic sufferer. On one occasion, I had prepared a large vegetable lasagne of wheat pasta, carrots, celery and water chestnuts, together with tomatoes, onions, green peppers, potatoes, and eggplant and I had planned to take the dish to a potluck gathering with friends. However, when this event was cancelled, I served the dish at home for several days in a row. As Ross thrived on the seemingly wholesome dish, I became more achy each day. My joints were hot, and I felt listless and depressed. I consulted my bookshelves and rediscovered Carlson Wade's book, *Inner Cleansing*, in which he states the dangers of the nightshade family of vegetables for those with osteoarthritis. As mentioned earlier, the nightshade family is made up of potatoes, peppers, eggplant and tomatoes (PPETs for short). These are the basic ingredients for vegetable lasagne, together with wheat pasta, which I later discovered I was also allergic to. I had unwittingly given myself a large dose of foods that were toxic to my system.

Toxic wastes can be stored anywhere in the body, not only around arthritic joint sites. They can accumulate in glands and can circulate throughout the bloodstream. There are several effective ways to eliminate these toxins. In *Inner Cleansing*, I found the following helpful guidelines:

- Pay careful attention to what the body is being asked to digest. Eat foods that not only do not increase toxins, but that actually help in the process of dissolving and washing away undesirable, pain-causing body wastes (these include raw vegetables, fruit, juices, and spring water; cod liver oil and salmon oil also help to soothe raw joints).
- Regular gentle massage is recommended to stimulate the muscles connected to joints and spinal vertebrae so that they release their toxins.
- Garlic, a natural anti-inflammatory, contains allisotin, used by body enzymes to wash away the wastes that cling to joints, muscles and related organs. It can add flavour to many dishes and should be used liberally in cooking.
- Simple stretching exercises before taking a baking soda bath prepare the way for further external release of toxins.

Detoxifying the system can begin with a simple regimen of fresh raw fruits and vegetables. For breakfast, I recommend a plate of fresh fruit in season. Chew well to aid the digestive process. Mid-morning, drink a glass of either freshly squeezed fruit or vegetable juice. For lunch, I suggest a plate of fresh, raw, seasonal vegetables, eaten at a leisurely pace and chewed well. Mid-afternoon, drink another glass of either fresh-fruit or vegetable juice. For the evening meal, I recommend another plate of different vegetables. Before retiring, take another glass of fresh vegetable juice. The high natural mineral content of the juice helps me to sleep. If I feel cold or shivery, I steam the vegetables and puree them with the water used to steam them. Plentiful fresh spring water should also be consumed to help flush out the loosened toxins, and warm herbal teas can be drunk at any time for flavour and comfort. I still follow this regimen for a day or two whenever I need it, and it quickly puts me back on track.

Another good approach is the Wild Rose Herbal detoxification program—a complete kit that can be purchased from a healthfood store. It includes an easy food plan that supports the program and does not leave me feeling deprived or unwell. I usually feel a bit headachy the first day until the flushing begins, then I feel progressively better, sleep better, have more energy and, of course, feel good about nurturing myself towards good health. I have also used the lemon and cayenne juice fasting technique described by Stanley Buroughs in his book, *The Master Cleanser*. This, too, is a gentle way of fasting. However, any dietary change works best when we know which fruits and vegetables are most suitable for our bodies.

These can be determined by a Vega Test at the office of a naturopathic physician. My first testing showed that I had very high levels of candida—an extremely common condition that occurs when the body has excessive yeast in the intestinal tract. A balance of yeast and bacteria in the colon is necessary for healthy digestion. I was given a list of foods to avoid, and was surprised to see that plums, lemons and grapes were not allowed. Prune juice with lemon slices in spring water had been my pre-dinner drink, since I no longer drank wine, and grapes had been my pick-me-up treat! I had also been eating homemade wheat germ muffins, before I discovered that I was allergic to all wheat substances. What I believed to be a healthy diet was actually increasing my discomfort.

I returned to the naturopathic clinic within a month of my first testing, and underwent the same testing procedure. My candida levels were down and, for the next month, they remained at that level. However, eating enough of the right foods was proving difficult, so I phoned the doctor's office, complaining of cold and hunger. Obviously this was a familiar complaint for patients at this level of the cleansing program, for the cheery voice that answered my call was instantly able to provide me with some allergy-free soup recipes, and the name of a baker who made delicious kamut and spelt breads. I returned for further testing a few weeks later, and was found to be completely clear of candida. As a result, several forbidden foods were allowed back into my diet. From a list of 109 foods tested, dairy products, shrimps, peanuts, chocolate, tomatoes, barley, wheat bran, yeast, wine and sugar were still not allowed. The foods most often found to be unsuitable for osteoarthritis sufferers are the ones most people tend to like very much, and are usually addictive, such as coffee, tea, chocolate, ice cream and sugar. In addition to the supplements I was already taking, it was suggested that I add Citricidal—a natural internal germicidal in tablet form, to be taken after each meal. I did not feel deprived on the diet, having found quite a few tasty food substitutes that I learned to cook with. The tests were very valuable in that they gave me information specific to my needs. As a result, I now have a tool that I can use to keep me in good health for the rest of my life.

Naturopathic physicians usually prescribe specialized detoxification programs to suit individual needs. It is recommended that cleansing programs be followed twice a year. Fasting programs can also be very beneficial but should be monitored by a health professional.

In 1992, when I felt the need for deeper internal cleansing, I learned that Evans Hermon, RN, whom I had known for many years, was offering a residential fasting/cleansing program at her home in Madeira Park on British Columbia's Sunshine Coast. The Holistic Fasting Retreat was held in the cozy hillside home of Evans and Jock Hermon. Evans is a registered nurse who teaches and practises many of the holistic healing arts. Since there are often emotional, as well as physical, changes occurring during the fast, the process requires the sensitivity and knowledge of well-trained people and should be done in a nurturing environment. I felt confident in Evans's ability and looked forward to this five-day retreat in the company of two other women.

I was given instructions (outlined below) on how to prepare myself by modifying my diet for three or four days at home, prior to the retreat. The purpose of this was to help my body move easily and comfortably through this gentle juice fast.

Transitional Diet

Early Morning: A glass of hot water with the juice of half a fresh lemon. Half an hour later, an apple or two.

Mid-morning: Another piece of fruit.

Between Meals: Drink as much pure water as possible.

Lunch: A green salad with as many different kinds of sprouts as possible. For a salad dressing, blend together some herbs (eg fresh basil, rosemary, and tarragon, with garlic), add 2 tbsp of pure water, ½ a peeled lemon and a ¼ cup of cold-pressed oil. A cereal product such as a muffin or a slice of rye bread or rice cracker should be included.

Mid-Afternoon: A piece of fruit, celery or carrot sticks.

Supper: Steamed vegetables and short-grain brown rice, or repeat lunch menu.

Herbal teas between meals but not during.

Upon my arrival at the Fasting Retreat, I was greeted warmly and shown to my room. The two other women and I were then given our first drink of the day—a liver cleanser made of garlic, orange juice, and flaxseed oil. Evans laughingly said that the only cup of coffee we would get this week would be used as a coffee enema—and so began our five days of internal cleansing. This was to be a significant turning point for me in dealing with and overcoming osteoarthritis.

Each day of our retreat, fresh fruit juices, wheat grass picked from the Evans' garden and juiced, delicious warm vegetable potassium broths, and comforting ginger tea were served. Between meals, we drank several glasses of cool spring water.

As the fast progressed, we enjoyed the restful leisure time to be by ourselves. We also had the choice of sharing with our companions the physical and emotional changes we were all experiencing. Each day brought releases from old emotional baggage. Our sense of well-being grew as we exercised, danced, laughed, cried, and walked in the evening stillness by the sea. Before going to bed, we climbed into the hot tub in the garden under the stars and watched clouds drift over the face of the moon. We began to feel cleansed and relaxed in body, mind and spirit.

On our last day, my companions and I decided not to break our fast. We felt so well that we wanted to continue with the juices and broth for a few more days at home. We would then return to the Transition Diet, and continue our new ways of eating and nurturing ourselves.

Traditions from India, China, Native America, and many other cultures recommend that all adults conduct an internal cleanse at regular intervals throughout their lives as a way of keeping in touch with the body's natural rhythms. This cleansing process nurtures the soul, for it is in these quiet times that we tap into the healing powers we all have within.

Enemas are a gentle way of washing out old fecal matter from the body, together with the toxins stored therein. Pre-prepared kits are available and can be used with warm water for home use (It is advisable to check with a naturopathic physician before using any of these methods.)

Colon therapy detoxifies and rids the entire colon of accumulated materials and toxins. This is done in a systematic way using water irrigation to help eliminate old impacted fecal matter. After making my dietary changes and undergoing the first stages of detoxification, colon irrigation was the next logical step in my healing process.

Colonic irrigation, in conjunction with a cleansing diet, herbs, and fibre, is the optimum way to remove toxins. I was familiar with taking enemas while fasting, but I was a bit unsure of a full colonic. However, I went to see a rosy-cheeked, healthy young woman named Carolyn who, through her own colonic experiences while battling cancer, had decided to train in this much-needed therapy. Her warm, private workroom, and her sensitive manipulation with speculum and hoses allowed me to completely relax. Releasing old toxic build-up left me feeling a little like a helium balloon. After each visit, I floated home to rest with a cup of warm herbal tea.

Hydrotherapy has long been known as an effective and natural way to wash out accumulated toxins from the body and bring relief from joint and muscle pain. In the winter of 1849, Father Sebastian Kneipp cured himself of tuberculosis of the lungs by daily plunging his body into the waters of the river Danube. He later wrote about this ancient method of healing in his famous book, *My Water Cure*. In 1886, his book was published and people came from far and wide, either to take his cure or to learn his techniques. Hydrotherapy uses water in all its forms—liquid, ice, or steam. Each form can bring about either internal or external cleansing to help balance the body.

Drinking six-to-eight glasses of pure spring water a day works as a natural stimulus to flush toxins from the body. Taking a sauna is a way of using moist heat to cause the pores of the skin to open and release toxins through perspiration. Inhaling vapours over a bowl of hot water containing a few drops of eucalyptus or friars balsam, with the head and the bowl draped in a towel, helps loosen congestion of the head and chest.

The most comforting form of hydrotherapy for the osteoarthritis sufferer is a good warm bath. Before immersing myself in the water, I use a long-handled bath brush to stimulate my body and to gently slough off dead skin. I remove the handle for the first part of the brushing. Then, with a gentle circular motion, I begin to brush from the toes on the right foot up the leg and around the buttocks. I repeat this process on the left side. I then do the same for the belly, hips, chest and breasts. Always working towards the heart, I progress to the fingertips of the each hand, brushing over and under and up the arm, and circling around the shoulder. Finally, I re-attach the long handle to the brush and vigorously scrub my spine. If hands, wrists and shoulders are too painful to grasp a bath brush, as mine were to begin with, there are stretchy nylon bath gloves with a crinkly surface that can be used instead.

When I am ready, I lower myself into a bath filled with comfortably hot water, which contains sea salt, baking soda, or Epsom salts. The addition of aromatherapy oils further relaxes the limbs that are now cushioned by the buoyancy of the water, allowing toxins to be released from sore muscles and joints. After relaxing for fifteen-to-twenty minutes, I release the water and, using either a hand spray or standing under the shower, rinse my body for about three minutes, gradually adjusting the temperature from comfortably hot to lukewarm. I get out of the bath slowly, pat my body dry with a warmed towel and get into bed with a cup of relaxing herbal tea.

Another form of hydrotherapy is a herbal wrap whereby a sheet or towel is soaked in hot water to which appropriate herbs have been added. The sheet is wrapped around the body and then covered with a warm blanket. While the body relaxes, the herbal wrap stimulates the release of toxins. When the undersheet appears dry, the body is given a warm water rinse and the usual comforting cup of herbal tea.

To stimulate poor circulation of feet and legs, while soothing varicose veins and helping to reduce swelling and discomfort, take a good warm bath, giving the toes and feet a rosy glow. After drying off, pull on a pair of cotton socks that have been soaked in very cold water, and then wrung out. Over these, pull on a pair of warm wool socks. Put on warm nightwear and hop into bed, wrapping the feet in a warm towel. Discard the socks when dry, and enjoy a wonderful night's sleep.

Chapter 5 / Finding the Right Foods

Wishing won't make it so,
but a transformed consciousness will.
Take back your life and be free.
—Dr Stuart Grayson, *Spiritual Healing*

The crippling disease of osteoarthritis can only be permanently and effectively conquered by rebuilding and restoring overall health. This means improving the function of the vital organs, enhancing glandular activity, and promoting optimal digestion and elimination.

Changing my diet was therefore one of the most important steps on my healing journey. It is hard to change any habit—especially where food is concerned—because it represents our first experience of being nurtured. However, discovering a holistic approach to new foods and ways of preparing them creates a sense of self-nurturing that eases the way through these changes.

Shopping for special breads, wheat-free pastas, selected fresh fruits and vegetables, and exploring the full range of non-dairy products gave buying, growing, and eating food a whole new dimension. I delighted in buying fruits, vegetables and eggs from a local organic farmer. His fresh produce was attractively laid out, with prices clearly marked on a blackboard. Having determined the cost of my purchases, I paid by the honour system, placing my money in a large open tin. As I drove homeward down the lane, I experienced a warm sense of well-being from nurturing myself with these wholesome foods.

Live foods formed an integral part of my new regimen. Foods that are 'alive' are those picked fresh from the garden or from an organic farm and processed immediately. Seeds that are sprouted in a glass jar sitting on top of the warm refrigerator are indeed alive and, in their sprouted state, contain more nourishment than in their dry form. Sprouting seeds in a corner of your kitchen is a delightful way to produce fresh green foods for winter salads. Sprouted seeds are a powerhouse of nutrition, containing protein, fats, B-complex vitamins, vitamin E, calcium, iron, phosphorus, potassium, and magnesium. Wheat berries, alfalfa, almonds, lentils, mung beans, sesame and sunflower seeds are the easiest to grow, and are also the best tasting. Ann Wigmore's *The Sprouting Book* provides all the information required by novice sprouters. In another of her books, *The Wheatgrass Book*, she describes the incredible healing properties of this extraordinary plant that she, in large part, brought to the attention of the public. I met Ann many years ago in Vancouver, BC, when she rode her bicycle to deliver her freshly squeezed, life-saving juices to her customers. Later, she moved to Boston where she founded the Ann Wigmore Foundation.

Juicing fruits and vegetables at home is strongly recommended as fresh juices provide an abundance of powerful nutrients. When buying a juicer, it is advisable to choose one with a slow masticating speed as it will produce more fibre, enzymes, vitamins and trace minerals and will give the most nourishing results. Many green vegetables, such as spinach, parsley, endive, and lettuce, can be added to celery, carrots, and beetroots to make a surprising variety of flavours. Most juicer manufacturers include recipes for fruit and vegetable cocktails, purees, relishes, muffins, cakes, breads, and ice cream in which fresh juices can be used. In some of these recipes, substitute fruits and vegetables may have to be found to suit your particular dietary needs.

Substitute Foods

There are many good books on special dietary needs. I used the following as an introduction to alternative foodstuffs, and for basic reference:

- *Fit for Life II—Living Health*, by Harvey & Marilyn Diamond.
- *Freedom from Allergy Cookbook,* by Ron Greenberg, MD, with Angela Nori.
- *Vegan Delights*, by Jeanne Marie Martin.
- *The Ayurvedic Cookbook*, by Amadear Morningstar, with Urmila Desai.
- *The Joy of Cooking*, by Irma Rambauer and Marion Rambauer Becker. This is an old standard, found in most kitchens, that gives basic cookery information.

Wheat Substitutes

My Vega test results prompted me to seek out the many 'rediscovered' grains that are invaluable to those who cannot eat wheat.

Kamut is an ancient grain that originated in the Mediterranean area thousands of years ago. It was used as early as 4000 BC in Egypt where it was referred to as the 'Grain of the Pharaohs.' Kamut is a good source of complex carbohydrate, protein, and amino acids, and has a higher mineral content than wheat. It has a sweet, nut-like flavour, and is good for bread-making.

Spelt is another ancient grain that was prominent in early medieval Europe. It contains more protein, fats and crude fibre than wheat, and has special carbohydrates that play a role in blood-clotting and stimulating the body's immune system. It is also more easily digested than wheat and its nutrients are therefore more readily absorbed.

Quinoa, another nutritious ancient grain, is high in protein and has an almost complete amino acid balance. I cook it and use it as I would rice, thoroughly rinsing it first and being careful to remove any bits of gravel, which often remain after harvesting.

Millet is high in vitamins and very alkaline. It can also be cooked and served as an alternative to rice. Cooked rice and millet, or puffed millet and kamut are easily digested as breakfast cereals. These can be served with rice milk, soy milk, or seed milk.

Kamut, spelt, rice and tapioca yeast-free breads are now readily available in healthfood stores, and most manufacturers of these grains also provide recipes. Athletes are now finding additional energy and vitality from spelt and kamut products. As pastas, these grains are especially good with a generous serving of sauce. However, individuals with a severe wheat allergy should add these new grains to their diet gradually as they could, possibly, react to them in the same way they react to wheat.

Also rediscovered this century were the writings of Hildegarde of Bingen, a Benedictine nun who lived in the middle ages (1098-1179). Her writing describes her basic spelt-flour diet which was rich in fibre and included chestnuts that, she says, are good for the brain, and galangal, a spice which is good for the heart. Similar in form to ginger root, galangal warms and balances the body. Information about her astonishing and diverse collection of books on healing sciences, poems, songs, and paintings, together with her famous Hildegarde Diet, can be found in *Hildegarde of Bingen's Medicine*, by Dr Wighard Strehlow and Gottfried Hertzka, MD.

Dairy Substitutes

Although not strictly a dairy substitute, the following blend is far healthier and, usually, better tolerated by most individuals than ordinary butter. Blend one pound of butter in one-and-a-half cups of cold-pressed virgin olive oil. This produces a flavoursome spread with more essential fatty acids than margarine or butter alone. It also has 50% less cholesterol and 50% less saturated fat than solid dairy butter. Keep in the refrigerator, taking serving portions to the table. My family has used this form of modified butter for many years for cooking and as a spread. The basic recipe is from Dr Adelle Davis's book, *Let's Get Well,* which suggests using soy, safflower, or peanut oils, but I prefer to use double virgin cold-pressed olive oil for its superior nutritional value.

Our bodies can tolerate these natural substances far better than the oils used in margarine. Recent research into trans fatty acids demonstrates that the hydrogenated oils used in margarine are injurious to our health. And the disturbing fact that dairy cows are being treated with chemicals, antibiotics and hormones is prompting many of us to make other choices. Herb-flavoured, pure cold-pressed olive oil, soybean oil, and flaxseed oil (never heated) can be drizzled on vegetables instead of butter.

Lecithin is another nutritious substance that can be used in numerous ways. As a fat emulsifier made from soy beans, it can be added to soups, fruit or vegetable salads, juices, gravies, sauces, dressings, hot or cold cereals and, in small amounts, to batter when baking. Soy lecithin spread has a butter-like consistency, but is dairy-free. It is made from soybean oil, soy lecithin, honey, soy flour, beta-carotene and salt.

As a milk substitute, commercial soy and rice milks may be blended together in equal proportions to improve the rather chalky taste of undiluted soy milk.

Soy yogurt can be used instead of dairy yogurt, and is good with fresh fruits and/or seeds added. The commercial varieties are sometimes sweetened with honey and they go well with fruits such as kiwis and peaches.

Another effective milk substitute is tofu powder, which can be reconstituted with water for use on cereals or as a drink. To make a soothing nighttime drink, stir one tablespoon of tofu powder and one tablespoon of finely ground almonds in a cup of warm water with a teaspoon of honey and a dash of nutmeg.

Cream Substitute

Blend the following ingredients for a surprisingly tasty alternative to regular cream:

1lb of firm silken tofu.
¼ cup of honey or maple syrup.
1 teaspoon of vanilla essence.
2 teaspoons of lemon juice.
2 teaspoons of grape seed oil.
Pinch of freshly grated nutmeg.

Keep refrigerated.

Cheese Substitutes

Soy cheese, made in the flavours of Cheddar, Mozzarella, and Italian White cheese, can be purchased as blocks or slices at most supermarkets these days. Parmesan-flavoured soy cheese is grated and can be used as a good substitute for regular Parmesan cheese. All these cheese substitutes will melt when cooked but their volume is not as great as that of regular cheeses.

Meat Substitutes

A commonly used meat substitute is dried textured soy protein which can be used in a variety of ways. This product is usually chicken- or bacon-flavoured with a light smoky taste. It can be added to grains, nuts, vegetables, used as a savoury filling, or made into burger-like patties.

Tofu is another versatile soybean product that can be used in sweet and savoury foods. An inexpensive source of protein, low in saturated fat, it comes in many forms: cheese, hamburger substitutes, chicken-flavoured niblets, artificial bacon pieces or even 'back bacon' slices.

Firm tofu can be marinated and used in casserole dishes, soups and quiches in place of meat. Medium-firm tofu can be crumbled and cooked as a scrambled egg substitute for those unable to eat eggs. Soft tofu can be used in desserts, mayonnaise and vegetable or fruit dips.

Sugar Substitutes

There are many sugar substitutes available, including organic maple sugar, honey, date sugar, and Sucanat, which is pure dried cane sugar juice that can be used for cookies and cakes. When replacing regular sugar in a recipe, try using one-third of a cup less than called for.

A very new form of sweetener is made from the Brazilian herb Stevia (which I tried growing in my garden, with little success). It is available in liquid, tablet and powder form for use in beverages and cooking.

Substitute Recipes

The following recipes are among those I adapted and modified to suit my changing needs over the years. What at first appeared to be a limited and dreary diet became, with a little creativity, an exciting way of preparing healthy food.

Nut Milks

Ingredients:

3 tbsp raw cashew nut pieces or blanched almonds
1 cup water

Method:

Thoroughly blend nuts with water until smooth.

Almond Milk Drink

Ingredients:

1 cup blanched almonds
4 cups pure spring water
maple syrup

Method:

Thoroughly blend nuts with water until smooth, adding a dash of maple syrup to taste.

Sunflower Seed Milk

Ingredients:

1 cup water
1/3 cup of ground sunflower seeds
2 or 3 pitted dates

Method:

Grind seeds in coffee grinder. Put in blender with water and blend. Pour liquid through a fine sieve.

Note: The same recipe can be used with sesame seeds.

Tofu Mayonnaise

Ingredients:

1lb firm tofu
1-1/2 cup raw ground cashew nuts
1/2 cup toasted cashew nuts ground
1/2 cup water with the juice of 1 lemon
1 tbsp honey
2 tbsp horseradish
1 green onion
dash of Braggs Liquid Aminos
dash of garlic powder
1/4 cup olive oil

Method:

Blend nuts water and lemon juice together. Add tofu, sweetener, horseradish and onion, Braggs Liquid Aminos, garlic powder, and blend together. Slowly add olive oil. Keep refrigerated.

Note: Braggs Liquid Aminos is a wheat-free, salt-free seasoning made from soybean concentrate.

Tofu Caesar Dressing

Ingredients:

5-6oz of soft tofu
2 tbsp lemon juice
1 tsp Dijon mustard
1/4 tsp anchovy paste (optional)
3 tbsp grated tofu Parmesan cheese
3 tbsp flaxseed or Udo's oil
Gomasio* and freshly ground pepper to taste

Method:

Blend all ingredients together. Dressing will keep, refrigerated, for up to two days. Toss with Romaine lettuce and top with croutons.

Note: Flaxseed oil spoils easily and must be refrigerated.

A tasty seasoning made from ground sesame seeds and sea salt. See recipe below.

Veggie Butter Dip

Ingredients:

1 cup modified butter
1 tbsp almond butter or tahini
1/2 tsp Gomasio
dash cayenne pepper
3 cups carrots and yam mixed
1 cup broccoli florets
1 clove garlic

Method:

Lightly steam vegetables. Put in blender, adding first four ingredients with a dash or two of Bragg's Liquid Aminos. Blend again. Keep chilled until served.

Nut and Seed Spread

Ingredients:

1 cup blanched ground almonds
1 cup ground sunflower seeds
1 medium carrot, finely grated
1 tbsp lemon juice
1/2 cup tofu mayonnaise
1/2 cup chopped parsley
2 garlic cloves
2 tbsp tamari
1 tsp cayenne pepper, marjoram, and Spike (a herbal salt sold in healthfood stores).

Method:

Soak nuts and seeds over night before blending ingredients in the order given. Chill and serve on soda bread, rye or rice crackers.

Gomasio

Ingredients:

2-1/4 cups ground toasted hulled sesame seeds
3/4 cup sea salt
1 tbsp sea kelp (I gather the deep rose-red dulse from the beach, and then dry and grind it)

Method:

Mix together. Keep well sealed. This salt adds a distinctive flavour to food, while lowering salt intake. Herbal salt may be made by finely grinding your favourite dried herbs, and adding them to Gomasio.

WHEAT-FREE BREADS

Soda Bread

Dry ingredients:

2 cups spelt flour
2 cups kamut flour
2 tbsp arrowroot
2 tsp baking powder
2 tsp baking soda
1 tsp salt
4 tbsp flaxseed, ground into a meal

Wet ingredients:

1-1/2 cups water
3 tbsp maple syrup
4 tbsp sunflower oil
2 tbsp apple cider vinegar
1/2 cups ground cashew nut pieces
1/2 cups ground sunflower seeds

Method:

Preheat oven to 375°F. Sift dry ingredients together. Blend wet ingredients with nuts and seeds. Slowly add wet to dry ingredients. As mixture stiffens, use hands to mix and knead for 2 minutes on flat surface. Shape loaf into a round and place on baking pan, or in a large bread pan that has been oiled and floured. Oil top of loaf. Bake 55-60 minutes.

Note: This recipe came from Jean Marie Martin's *Vegan Delight* and was modified to suit me. This bread helped me to not feel deprived in the early years of changing my diet—as did many of her recipes. I found most alternative flours required a little more liquid than did wheat flour.

Gabriele's Banana Bread

Ingredients:

2 ripe mashed bananas
2 eggs
1/2 cup oil
3/4 cup Sucanat
1-1/4 cups spelt flour
1 tsp baking soda and dash of salt
1/2 cup chopped walnuts

Method:

Beat bananas and eggs, and add oil. Add Sucanat, flour, soda, salt and nuts, in that order. Pour into loaf pan and bake for a good hour at 350°F.

Corn Bread

Ingredients

1 cup corn meal
3/4 cup spelt flour
1/4 cup corn flour
3 tsp baking powder
3/4 tsp salt
4 tbsp melted modified butter
2 tbsp corn syrup
1 cup mixed soy and rice milk
1 egg

Method:

Sift together all dry ingredients. Beat egg with milk, corn syrup, and melted butter. Stir liquid into dry ingredients. Pour into 8"x 8" pan or small loaf tin. Bake at 350°F for 20-25 minutes until lightly brown around edges.

Basic Spelt Muffins

Ingredients:

2-1/4 cups spelt flour
1 tbsp baking powder
1/2 tsp salt
1-1/4 cups milk (nut, seed or soy)
3 eggs beaten
2 tbsp sunflower oil

For sweet muffins add:
1/2 cup chopped nuts
1/2 cup chopped dates or raisins
1/4 cup honey
For savoury muffins add:
1/2 cup chopped pumpkin seeds
1/2 tsp garlic powder
1 tsp parsley
1/2 tsp thyme
1/2 tsp chervil

Method:

Preheat oven to 425ºF. Oil and flour muffin pans. Combine wet and dry ingredients, adding either the sweet or savoury ingredients. Mix until moistened. Fill pan 2/3 full with batter and bake for 17 minutes until brown. Serve savoury muffins with a slice of soy cheese or chutney spread.

Note: Taken from Dr Wighard Strephlow's booklet, *The Wonderful Spelt*, Purity Foods Inc., 2871 W. Jolly Rd, Okemos, MI 48864.

Currant or Blueberry Pancakes

Ingredients:

1-1/2 cup spelt flour or oat and millet flour mix
1/4 tsp salt
1 tbsp baking powder
1 egg
1 tbsp honey
1-3/4 cups orange juice
1 cup fruit

Method:

Combine wet and dry ingredients. Drop batter into hot skillet from a large spoon to form rounds. Flip when bubbles come to the surface and cook until lightly golden.

Note: As an alternative to these pancakes, healthfood stores often sell Toaster Waffles, which are wheat-, gluten-, egg-, and dairy-free. Spread waffles with strawberry conserve, red currant jelly, or banana slices. Top with tofu cream.

SOUPS

Cold Day Broth

Ingredients:

8 cups of water
2 tsp salt or Gomasio
1 medium parsnip in chunks
2 large carrots in chunks
2 celery stalks
2 green onions
handful of mushrooms, halved
1 tsp turmeric and dash of pepper

Method:

Combine everything in soup pot. Bring to boil, reduce heat and simmer for 1 hour. Cool, strain, and discard vegetables. This broth is great with soda bread and Seed and Nut spread.

Cauliflower Soup

Ingredients:

1/2lb cauliflower heads
1 clove garlic
1/2 cup hot apple juice
1 cup hot water
1/3 cup sunflower seeds
Spike to taste

Method:

Steam cauliflower for 8 minutes. Use one cup of steamer water and sunflower seeds, blend until liquefied to make milk. Add a handful of fresh herbs (sweet cicely, chives and gingermint) and blend again. Add the hot apple juice, cauliflower and Spike. Blend until smooth. Put in pan with 1 tsp butter and reheat gently. Do not boil.

Cream of Broccoli Soup

Ingredients:

4 cups washed broccoli flowerets
2 cloves garlic
1/2 cup sunflower seeds
1 tsp Braggs Liquid Aminos
Spike and pepper to taste
2 cups hot water

Method:

Steam broccoli 5 minutes. Blend 1/2 cups sunflower seeds in 1/2 cup hot steamer water until smooth. Add the other 1-1/2 cups hot water with the broccoli and garlic. Blend until thick and creamy. Taste; if needed add a pinch or two of oregano.

Note: Adapted from the *Ayurvedic Cookbook*.

Parsnip and Apple Soup

Ingredients:

2 tbsp coconut butter
1 medium onion
2 medium parsnips
1 medium cooking apple
2-1/4 cups vegetable stock
2 tbsp chopped parsley
1/2 tsp mixed dried herbs
2-1/4 cups milk: almond, cashew, sunflower seed or soy milk
salt and pepper to taste

Method:

Chop vegetables and apples and sauté in pan with coconut butter, stirring until onion is transparent. Add stock and herbs. Bring to boil. Reduce heat and cover, and simmer 25-30 minutes. Add milk. Blend soup in small quantities. Reheat gently to serving temperature. Season to taste.

Note: Non-hydrogenated coconut oil contains 'good' fat and does not elevate the bad cholesterol level (LDL). It adds a wonderful subtle flavour to foods.

Lima Bean and Rice Soup

Ingredients:

1/4 cup cooked Basmati rice
1/2 cooked lima beans
2 tbsp grape seed or sunflower seed oil
1/2 tsp mustard seeds
1/2 turmaric
2 cups chopped carrots and yams
1 celery stalk
4 cups water
2 tsp corriander powder
1 tsp Gomasio or sea salt
1/4 cups frozen peas

Method:

In saucepan, heat oil, add mustard seeds. When they pop, add turmeric and carrots. Cook 3-4 minutes. Add rice, beans, celery and water, coriander and Gomasio. Boil 15 minutes over medium heat. Add peas at the last minute. Serve hot.

Note: Modified from the *Ayurvedic Cookbook*. I replaced green peppers with celery to avoid the nightshade family of vegetables (potatoes, peppers, eggplants, and tomatoes), which are unsuitable for many people.

SALADS

Quinoa Salad

Ingredients:

1-1/2 cups well washed quinoa
2 cups water
6 green onions
1 clove garlic finely chopped
2-3 cups chopped parsley
1/4 cup mint and fresh basil leaves chopped
1 tomato skinned and seeded
1/2 cup olive oil
1 tsp flaxseed oil
Braggs Liquid Aminos and cayenne pepper, to taste

Method:

Cook and cool the quinoa. Add all the other ingredients but the tomato and toss. Before serving, dice the tomato, add to basil and use as a garnish on salad bowl.

Note: For tomato-sensitive people, this vegetable, which is used only as a garnish, can be easily removed. For those who can tolerate a small amount of some 'forbidden foods,' this is a way to re-introduce them. Check with your Vega Testing Clinic. A Four-day Rotation Plan is discussed in the *Freedom from Allergy Cookbook*. It is now possible for me to re-introduce previously forbidden foods without discomfort by observing my own rotation plan. Discretion is the watchword!

Beetroot Salad with Horseradish

Ingredients:

2 medium-sized peeled and grated beetroots
2 large carrots, grated
2 chopped green onions
1/2 cup chopped pumpkin seeds (lightly toasted)

Dressing:

1 tbsp creamed horseradish
4 tbsp soy yogurt
1/2 Spike (herb salt)
1-1/2 tsp date sugar or Sucanat

Method:

Pour dressing over vegetables. Toss together and sprinkle seeds on top. Makes 2-3 servings.

Celery, Cucumber and Grape Salad

Ingredients:

4 celery sticks
1/2 English (long) cucumber
1-1/4 cups red grapes

Dressing:

1/2 cup tofu mayonnaise
1 tsp Dijon mustard
1/4 tsp ground nutmeg

Method:

Chop celery, peel cucumber in a stripe pattern and slice thinly. Halve grapes and remove seeds. Put all ingredients in salad bowl. Mix together with dressing. Season with sea salt and cayenne, and chill before serving.

Alfalfa Salad

Ingredients:

4 cups sprouted alfalfa
1 cup mung bean sprouts

Piquant Dressing:

3/4 cup apple cider vinegar
1/2 cup water
2 tbsp chopped chives
2 tsp sweetener
1 tsp paprika (if tolerated)
2 tsp tahini
1/2 tsp Gomasio
1/2 tsp Dijon mustard

Blended together, makes about 2-1/2 cups

Method:

Mix all green sprouts together and toss with dressing.

Note: Modified from *Crank's Recipe Book.*

SAVOURIES, SAUCES & PASTRY CRUSTS

Potato Frittata

Ingredients:

2 cups cooked diced potatoes (or yams)
1 chopped onion
3/4 cups diced marinated tofu, lightly browned with the onion
5 eggs
1/2 cup grated soy cheese
1/4 cup soy and rice milk mix
1/2 cup tofu mayonnaise
salt and pepper, paprika (or nutmeg)

Method:

Heat oven to 350°F. Oil a 9" or 10" quiche plate. Place potatoes/yams, onions and tofu in plate. Whisk together eggs, milk, mayonnaise and seasonings. Pour over potato/tofu mixture. Sprinkle with cheese, paprika or nutmeg. Bake for 30 minutes until eggs are set. Serves 6.

Tofu Marinade

Ingredients:

1lb organic firm tofu, washed and well drained
1/4 cup olive oil
4 sliced mushrooms
2 green onions chopped
1/2 inch finely grated ginger root
1/2 cup apple juice with a dash of sherry
1/4 cup Tamari, pinch of cloves, Gomasio and freshly ground pepper

Method:

Warm oregano in frying pan until aromatic. Add oil, green onions, mushrooms and ginger, stirring until soft and blended. Pour in apple juice, sherry and tamari. Simmer, adding Gomasio and freshly ground pepper to taste. Allow sauce to come up to boiling. Remove from heat and pour marinade over sliced or cubed tofu. Keep marinated tofu in refrigerator overnight.

Salmon Loaf with Dulse

Ingredients:

1oz dried dulse
1/2 cup nut milk or whole soy milk
3/4 cup fine spelt breadcrumbs
3 eggs just stirred with a fork
juice of a 1/2 lemon
1 tbsp chopped parsley
1 tbsp chopped chives and dash of ground fennel seeds
1 tsp Gomasio
1 16oz can salmon

Method:

Crumble the dulse finely. Warm milk and mix in breadcrumbs and dulse. Mix all other ingredients together. Use grape seed or corn oil inside Pyrex loaf pan. Fill with salmon mixture. Bake for 1 hour at 350°F. Serve hot or cold with tofu mayonnaise, to which fresh minced parsley has been added.

Nutty Millet and Basmati Rice Pilaf

Ingredients:

2 tbsp olive oil
1 medium onion, minced
1 cup Basmati rice, rinsed
1/2 cup hulled millet
1-3/4 cup water
1/3 cup boiling water
1/2 cup green peas
1/2 cup walnut pieces

Method:

Heat oil in medium-sized saucepan, add onion and sauté until soft and transparent, about 2 minutes. Add Basmati rice and millet, stir until lightly toasted and golden in colour. Add 3/4 the water and bring to a boil. Lower heat, cover, and cook for 30 minutes. Stir, then add 1/3 cup boiling water. Cover and cook over very low heat for 15 more minutes. Remove from heat, add green peas, then stir well. Return pan to stove and cook for another 5 minutes over low heat, add nuts, and toss. Serves 4.

Note: This recipe was taken from *Sam Okomoto's Incredible Vegetables*, an unusual collection of recipes that blends the principles of good nutrition with traditional Asian cuisine and popular Western-style cooking.

Beetroot and Rice Loaf

Ingredients:

1 large onion
1 large carrot
1 medium rutabaga turnip
1 medium zucchini
1 large yam
2 medium beetroots
2 garlic cloves
1/3 cup coconut butter
1/2 cup sunflower seeds
1 tsp each of ground cumin, dried dill and tarragon
1/2 tsp sea salt (Gomasio)
1 tsp pepper (cayenne)
1 1/2 cooked brown rice.

Method:

Chop vegetables in food processor and sauté in coconut butter until limp. Add mixture to seeds, herbs and cooked rice. Press into a loaf pan covered with foil and bake for 1 hour. Uncover and bake for a further 30 to 45 minutes. Toothpick test for doneness. Slice on serving platter and serve with carrot sauce.

Carrot Sauce

Ingredients:

2 cups chopped onions
2 cups sliced carrots
1/4 cup light olive oil
2-1/2 cups vegetable stock
1/2 cup toasted pumpkin seeds
1 tsp dried basil

Method:

Sauté onion and carrots in oil until brown. Add vegetable stock and cook until carrots are tender, and the water is somewhat reduced. Pour some liquid from pan into blender, add pumpkin seeds and blend. Gradually add all the carrots, onions and stock and blend until smooth. Add dash of salt, pepper and allspice to taste.

Note: As an alternative to vegetable stock, use previously saved vegetable steamer water to which 1 tbsp dried onion soup powder has been added.

Curried Split Peas

Ingredients:

1 cup green split peas, soaked overnight
1 medium onion, chopped
2 medium carrots, chopped
4 tbsp modified butter
2 medium cooking apples, chopped
1 tbsp curry powder
3 tbsp spelt, kamut or rice flour
1/3 cup soaked raisins
1 cup coconut milk
salt and pepper to taste
1/4 cup toasted coconut
1 tbsp chopped parsley

Method:

In saucepan, cover peas with water and bring to boil. Simmer covered for 1/2 hour. Remove from heat and keep to one side. Melt modified butter in a skillet and sauté vegetables. Add apples. Mix curry powder with flour and stir into vegetables. Now drain the peas, reserving 1 cup of cooking liquid. Add split peas and liquid to the pan with remaining ingredients. Bring gently to a boil, reduce heat, and simmer about 1/2 hour. Season to taste. Serve over cooked rice. Sprinkle with toasted coconut and minced parsley.

Lentil Cheese Wedge

Ingredients:

1 cup red lentils
2 cups water
1 large onion
2 tbsp modified butter
1 1/2 cups grated soy cheese
1 tsp mixed herbs or summer savoury
1 egg
1 cup spelt or kamut breadcrumbs
2oz sunflower seeds
1 tbsp minced parsley

Method:

Cook lentils in water until soft and liquid has been absorbed. Chop onion. Melt modified butter in saucepan and sauté onion. Combine all the ingredients together and press into an oiled 9" pie pan. Bake at 375°F for 30 minutes or until brown. Dust generously with soy Parmesan cheese and parsley. This dish is great for picnics and potluck dinners.

Smoked Cheese and Spinach Pie

Ingredients:

1 uncooked pie shell
1 tbsp Dijon mustard
3/4 cup grated tofu cheddar cheese
1/2 cup of TSP (textured soy protein) smoked bacon bits
2 cups washed and chopped spinach
1 tbsp olive oil
1 cup sliced mushrooms
2 tsp Braggs Liquid Aminos
3 eggs
1 cup nut, rice or full soy milk
1/2 cup thick almond milk
1 tsp corn flour

Method:

Brush uncooked pie shell with Dijon mustard and sprinkle with cheeses. Sauté mushrooms in oil, then add Braggs Liquid Aminos. Add spinach and cook until soft. Spread mushrooms, spinach and bacon bits on top of the cheese. Beat eggs and milks together, adding corn flour. Pour over vegetables. Bake at 425°F for 15 minutes. Lower heat to 300°F. Continue baking for 20-30 minutes until a knife inserted comes out clean. Dust with soy Parmesan cheese. (Soy cheese does not rise as much as other cheeses.)

Note: Adapted from a recipe in *The Tassajara Recipe Book,* which is used at the Zen Mountain Centre, San Francisco. The book contains the Centre's 'Favourites of the Guest Season,' in addition to beautiful verses that remind us to cook mindfully and lovingly, for we nourish the soul as well as the body.

Spiced Chick Pea Patties

Ingredients:

1 19oz can chick peas
1 egg
3 tbsp chopped parsley
2 crushed garlic cloves
1 tsp ground cumin
1 tsp basil
1/2 tsp turmeric
dash of salt, pinch of cayenne

Coating: Beaten egg and rice flour

Method:

Mash peas, reserving 3 tbsp liquid to add with the herbs and spices. Form mixture into eight patties. Dip in beaten egg then in rice flour. Fry in coconut butter or oil of your choice. When golden brown, drain on paper towels and serve.

Basic White Sauce

Ingredients:

2 cups thick nut, seed, or soy milk
2-1/2 tbsp corn flour
2 tbsp modified butter, melted in pan
cayenne pepper and sea salt to taste

Method:

Beat all the ingredients together in order given. Stir over medium heat until sauce thickens. Remove from heat immediately and serve.

Cheese Sauce

Ingredients:

To Basic White Sauce, add:
1 tsp Dijon mustard
1 cup soy cheddar cheese
soy Parmesan cheese to taste
freshly grated pepper

Method:

Heat and serve as soon as cheese melts

Curry Sauce

Ingredients:

To Basic White Sauce, add:
1-1/2 tsp curry powder mixed to a thin paste with apple juice
1 tbsp of spicy chutney that has raisins in it
1 egg

Method:

Put all ingredients in the blender and begin blending. Add 1 egg and blend until smooth (you may need to thin with a little more nut milk). Return to saucepan and gently bring to serving temperature.

Fish Sauce

Ingredients:

To Basic White Sauce, add:
2 tsp of ground fennel seed
1 tbsp sherry
1 tbsp minced parsley

Heat and serve.

Nut Gravy

Ingredients:

1 cup toasted cashew milk
1 cup seed or soy milk
2 tbsp chopped onion
2 tbsp corn flour
1 tbsp Braggs Liquid Aminos or Miso
2 tbsp chopped chives
2 tbsp oil

Method:

Sauté onion in oil. Mix corn flour into nut milk and add Braggs Liquid Aminos. Pour into the onion mixture and cook to thicken. Add chopped chives, and serve.

Pastry Crust Substitute

Ingredients:

1 cup spelt flour
1/2 cup rice flour
2 tsp baking powder
2 tbsp oil
1/2 cup water

Method:

Sift flour and baking powder together. Add oil and water mix. With fingers, spread pizza base into a 9" oiled pie plate. Pat out to an even ¼" thickness.

Vegetable Pizza

Topping for Pastry Crust Substitute:

1 tsp horseradish cream
1/2 cup thinly sliced onions
1/2 cup thinly sliced zucchini
1/2 cup thinly sliced mushrooms
2 cups grated soy Italian white cheese
2 tbsp powdered soy Parmesan cheese
1 tbsp dried basil leaves or chopped fresh leaves
1/4 cup chopped walnuts or pecans

Method:

Rub pizza base lightly with horseradish cream. Spread onions, zucchini and mushrooms, and scatter with chopped basil leaves and walnuts. Top with 2 cups grated soy Italian white cheese. Bake at 425°F for about 24 minutes. Dust well with soy Parmesan cheese.

Almond Pie Crust

Ingredients:

1 cup blanched almonds
1/3 cup raisins
2 tbsp tahini or almond butter
2 tsp vanilla

Method:

Chop all ingredients in food processor until paste forms. Scrape sides and chop again. Use wet fingers to spread in 8" or 9" pie plate. Bake at 250° F. for 30 minutes. Cool before filling with glazed fruits, apples, peaches, or blue berries. Serve with tofu cream.

Spelt Flour Crust (rolled)

Ingredients:

2 cups spelt flour
1 tbsp rice flour
2 tsp baking powder
pinch of salt
6 tbsp sunflower seed oil
4 tbsp cold water
1 tbsp lemon juice

Method:

Mix dry ingredients in bowl. Whisk oil, water and juice and add to dry ingredients. Work together to make a manageable dough. Roll out between 2 sheets of wax paper. Bake at 415°F for 10 minutes. Lower heat to 350°F until brown.

Millet Pastry Crust

Ingredients:

1-1/2 cups millet flour
1/2 cup rice flour
1/2 cup modified butter
2 tsp baking powder
8 tbsp cold water
1 tbsp lemon juice

Method:

Mix in food processor. Knead dough on floured board. Press into oiled 8" or 9" pie pan. Prick with fork, and cover with wax paper and handful of beans to keep crust from rising. Bake at 420°F for 10 minutes. Take out wax paper and beans and reduce oven temperature to 350°F for another 15-20 minutes. Watch edge of pan as millet flour browns quickly. This makes 2 single piecrusts.

Coconut Crust

Ingredients:

1/2 cup melted modified butter
2 cups Angel flake coconut
fresh sliced strawberries

Method:

Combine butter and coconut and press evenly into an ungreased 8" or 9"pie plate. Bake 300°F for 20-35 minutes. Fill with sliced fresh strawberries and top with coconut milk custard.

Basic Custard Sauce

Ingredients:

3 tbsp vanilla custard powder
2-1/2 cups of nut, seed, soy or coconut milk
1 tsp modified butter
2 tbsp Sucanat

Method:

Stir custard powder into 1 cup of milk. Heat remaining milk, adding butter, and slowly bring to the boil. Stir into custard powder and milk mix, adding Sucanat. Return to pan and cook until thickened. This makes quite a stiff custard. For a pouring sauce, blend 1 cup of basic sauce with thick nut milk, and thin as needed.

Tofu Fruit Dessert

Ingredients:

1 tbsp agar agar
1/4 cup cold water
1 tbsp modified butter
3 tbsp ground cashew nuts or almonds
1 cup hot water
5oz (or 1/2 package of soft almond-flavoured tofu)
1lb sliced fresh strawberries

Method:

Mix agar agar in cold water to form a paste. Gradually add boiling water. When jelly-like, stir in modified butter. Set aside. Put ground nuts and hot water in blender and blend until smooth. Add agar agar mixture and blend. Add tofu and blend. Gradually add sweetener, vanilla and strawberries and blend until thick. Add 5 drops of angostura bitters (optional). Pour into dessert glasses, top with piece of whole fruit and chill. Other fresh fruits such as bananas, apricots and mangoes can be used. This mixture can be poured into an 8" pan over a coconut crust, chilled overnight and served with tofu cream.

Carob Squares

Ingredients:

4 tbsp melted butter
1 cup spelt flour
1/2 tsp baking soda
1 tsp baking powder
pinch of salt
1/4 cup Sucanat
1 egg, beaten, with 8oz nut, seed, or soy milk
1 tsp vanilla
4 tbsp carob powder
handful of almond flakes

Method:

Mix carob powder into modified butter. Make a well in sifted dry ingredients. Add carob mixture and vanilla. Slowly add egg and milk, beating well. Pour into 8" x 8" oiled pan. Top with almond flakes. Bake 350°F for 30 minutes. Cool and cut into squares.

Note: Adapted from my friend Cicely's Four-minute Chocolate Cake recipe. When she and I had stayed too long painting together, we would race home to make this four-minute life-saver!

Agaba's Seed and Nut Cookies

Ingredients:

3oz modified butter
1 egg
2 tbsp. Sucanat
1/2 cup nut milk
1 cup spelt flour
1 tsp baking powder
1/2 tsp nutmeg
1/2 ground ginger
1/3 cup sesame seeds
1/3 cup chopped sunflower seeds
1/3 cup chopped and toasted sunflower seeds
1/3 cup sliced almonds
1/3 cup currants

Method:

Beat together butter, Sucanat and egg. Mix dry ingredients and milk alternately, adding seeds nuts and currants. Drop by tablespoonfuls on cookie sheet. Bake at 375°F for 15 minutes.

Date Squares

Ingredients:

3 cups oatmeal
1/2 cup rice flour
1/2 kamut flour
1/2 cup modified butter
1/4 cup honey
dash of salt
1/2 cup sunflower seeds chopped

Filling:

1/2lb chopped dates
1-1/2 cups water
1 tbsp lemon juice
1 tbsp ground orange peel

Method:

To make crust, rub butter into flour, stir in honey, add salt, seeds and oatmeal. For filling, cook dates and spices until liquid is absorbed. Oil and flour a 9" x 9" pan. Spread half the oatmeal mixture in the pan, pressing lightly. Bake at 350°F for 15 minutes. Remove from oven and spread the hot date mixture over the crust. Spread the remaining oat and flour mixture evenly over the filling. Bake for another 15-20 minutes until lightly brown. Delicious served warm with chilled silken tofu cream.

Tofu Cream

1 349g package of Mori-Nu Lite Extra firm silken-style tofu
1/4 cup honey/maple syrup
1 tsp vanilla essence
2 tsp lemon juice.

Method:

Blend all ingredients until thick and creamy. Use as a delicious topping for desserts.

Chocolate Mousse Pudding

Blend half of the tofu cream with 1/2-3/4 cup of pure Dutch cocoa powder. Then add the other half of the tofu cream and blend well. Pour into chocolate cups and chill for four hours. Before serving, garnish with chopped toasted almonds.
This is my favourite healthy, delicious dessert.

Note: After experimenting with various wheat flour substitutes, I found the following flour mix to be the most acceptable—even among those who do not have wheat allergies:

1kg of organic spelt flour
1 cup oat flour
1 cup of non-fat soy flour
1 cup of sweet rice flour

Bon appétit!

71

Chapter 6 / Supplements, Herbs & Other Natural Remedies

All strength, all healing of every nature
is the changing of the vibrations from within—
the attuning of the divine within the living tissue of a body to
Creative Energies. This alone is healing.
Whether it is accomplished by the use of drugs,
the knife or what not, it is the attuning of the living
cellular force to its spiritual heritage.

—Edgar Cayce, quoted in Dr Harold Reilly's book,
Handbook for Drugless Therapy

Like many naturopathic physicians and other healthcare practitioners concerned about the widespread use of anti-inflammatory drugs, I had my own misgivings. These were confirmed by the words of Dr McDougall, in his book, *The McDougall Program: Twelve Days to Dynamic Health*:

A recent study has shown that popular non-steroidal, anti-inflammatory arthritis drugs, which inhibit the activity of the hormones called prostaglandins, can actually cause osteoarthritis to progress more quickly, destroying more joint tissue than would be lost without the medication. Examples of prostaglandin-inhibiting drugs include aspirin, Indocin, Meclomen, Mortrin, Nalfon, Naprosyn, Rufen and Tolectin.

This information further convinced me of the need to find natural, holistic approaches to pain management. As a family, we had taken vitamin supplements for years. Now, with evidence of considerable bone loss in my wrists, I needed to add supplements for rebuilding bone and connective tissue.

When using supplements, herbs, and other natural remedies, it is important to find a holistic balance for each phase of recovery. For example, the green-lipped mussel painkiller that initially gave me great relief, became less effective after a period of time (I subsequently discovered, through Vega testing, that it contained a substance I was allergic to).

The following supplements are recommended as a general guideline, and the specific dosages for each individual would need to be determined by a healthcare practitioner:

Supplements

Vitamin A A soluble oil. The main sources are fish and fish liver oils. Salmon oil is now being offered in capsule form, in addition to halibut oil.

Vitamin B The B complex group of vitamins needs to be taken collectively, and in a balanced form. All Bs act synergistically; in other words, they need to exist simultaneously in the body in order to be effective. It is therefore important to find a complex that contains Vitamin B1 (Thiamine), B2 (Riboflavin), B5 (Pantothenic Acid), and B6 (Pyridoxine)—an important aid in stress relief. B12 is also essential as it prevents anemia. Brewers yeast is an excellent food source of B vitamins, but should be taken in gradually increasing amounts as can be tolerated (it should not be taken by those suffering from a candida overgrowth).

A balanced B complex tablet also includes minerals in its formula, such as choline and inositol, plus chelated minerals of calcium, potassium, iron, magnesium, manganese, zinc, copper, iodine, chromium and selenium, together with non-medical ingredients to aid in assimilation. Iron-free B Complex tablets are also available.

Vitamin C A factor in the maintenance of bones, cartilage, teeth and gums. I use a natural compound of rosehips, rutin, hesperidin, bioflavonoids and acerola.

Vitamin D This is the sunshine vitamin, attainable from the sun's rays and also found in milk. I do not drink milk, but I like to sunbathe for brief periods.

Vitamin E The natural form of this antioxidant is called d'alpha Tocopherol, and I take it with selenium, another powerful antioxidant that can be used internally, or externally for healing skin tissue.

Calcium Best taken at night with **magnesium**, **potassium** and **zinc**. Calcium is an important supplement for rebuilding bone tissue. I prefer a ratio of one part calcium to one-and-a-half parts magnesium. Adding a capsule of magnesium citrate enhances assimilation.

Garlic oil   Available in capsules or coated tablets. A natural lubricator, blood cleanser, and anti-bacterial and anti-fungal agent.

Lecithin   A fat emulsifier made from soybeans. It comes in granules, liquid or capsules. I use granules mixed together with equal amounts of freshly ground flaxseeds. Both substances should be kept refrigerated in a sealed glass jar. I grind a jarful of flaxseeds every few days and sprinkle them, with the lecithin, on my morning millet and rice, or on fruit moistened with soy or rice milk. I use liquid lecithin in baking. Lecithin and flaxseed oil also come in capsule form.

Milk Thistle   Supports liver detoxification. Comes in gelatin capsules.

Silica   Helps rebuild strong bones, teeth and hair. Available in gelatin capsule form. Gel-Silica Serves the same function as its plant sister, but is derived from quartz crystal. Small particles are suspended in liquid. Taken in juice, it is considered to be absorbed faster and more completely. It makes a great beauty mask too!

Chlorella   A natural green single-cell algae, containing amino acids and many other beneficial supplements. Available in small tablet form. In gelatin capsules, Chlorella is teamed with Carotenoid and Spirulina. I take these on alternate days. In the final stages of my recovery, I began using Super Blue Green Algae. This remarkable food supplement is harvested from the organic algae ponds at Klamath Falls, Oregon.

Alfalfa   A digestive aid in tablet form.

Citricidal   An intestinal cleanser made from grapefruit seed extract, supplied in tablet or liquid form, to be taken after meals. (Note: for sore throats, liquid Citricidal can be used as a gargle; 5-6 drops in 4oz water can be taken 3 times a day.)

Digestive enzymes   Scientific studies have revealed that digestive enzymes work as well as prescription non-steroidal anti-inflammatory drugs (NSAIDS) to control the pain of osteoarthritis. According to the *Clinical Drug Investigation* [19(1): 15-23, 2000], pain can be relieved within three weeks of using over-the-counter proteolytic digestive enzyme supplements (those that break down undigested protein), containing bromelain, trypsin and rutin.

Later, I added the following antioxidants to my supplement list: **Co-enzyme Q10**, **selenium** and **zinc**. Antioxidants inhibit free radicals, which are damaged oxygen molecules, attributed to increasing air pollutants, hydrogenated oils, deep-fried foods, ultra violet light, and thinning of our ozone layer. I also added **Glucosamine** with **Chondroitin Sulfate** for the joints, as well as **cayenne** for digestion, and **milk thistle** to cleanse the liver.

Natural Pain Relievers

Green-Lipped Mussel   I read a story in an Australian publication called *Nature and Health Journal*, describing research into the green-lipped mussel. This natural painkiller is suitable for arthritic conditions. I wrote to the magazine and was informed that this substance was soon to be released in the USA. Eventually it came to our local healthfood store and was one of my first alternative drug-free painkillers. It is available in capsule form.

Willow Bark This is a natural pain reliever, the forerunner of ASA Aspirin without the stomach discomfort that comes with long and continual use of ascetylsalicylic acid.

Devil's Claw Root A herbal anti-inflammatory in tablet form. I use this with great success.

Traumeel A homeopathic sublingual herbal preparation for pain, available in tablet form.

Tiger Balm Another natural soother for inflamed joints.

CamoCare Pain-Relieving Cream An ointment made with menthol and camphor in Chamomile. The Levomenol in this herb penetrates and soothes the skin. The smallest amount gently stroked into wrists and elbows brings almost immediate relief. Chamomile has long been used as nature's tranquillizer. Made popular by Victorian ladies who sipped its fragrant tea from wide, shallow, dainty cups—all the better to inhale Chamomile's soothing vapours.

Herbs

As a child, I was intrigued by the pungent smell of the herbs growing in our garden. I was taught to cook, dry, and store them. My knowledge and early use of herbs in alleviating common disorders expanded during my training at the Holistic Health Institute. Many years later, in the early 1980s, I became a student of Ella Birzneck, MH, one of the founders of the Dominion Herbal College of British Columbia.

Elderberry & cranberry juice

To make this blend, wash 100g of dried elderberries and add to 40 fluid ounces of cranberry juice, together with a 2-inch piece of galangal root. Simmer very gently for about an hour. After the berries have been reduced to a robust, dark liquid, strain and bottle, allowing the juice to cool before storing it in the refrigerator. Elderberries are a gentle detoxifier, cranberry juice is a mild diuretic, and galangal warms and balances the body. I fill a wineglass half-full with the juice, and top it up with either hot water or cool spring water for a healthy, pre-dinner drink.

Swedish Bitters

This is an elixir I make from pre-mixed, packaged herbs available in healthfood stores. I use it as an over-all tonic. I macerate the herbs in a jar of Chinese Ginseng brandy, and place the jar on a windowsill to be warmed by the sun. The jar is tipped and rolled daily for 14 days. This is racked off (strained) through gauze, bottled and well sealed. When needed, I take 1 tablespoon in 3/4 of a glass of warm water before breakfast as a morning pick-me-up. The original Swedish Bitters recipe is attributed to Swedish physician Dr Samtz, and can be found in Maria Treben's book, *Health through God's Pharmacy*. This book, a long-time favourite herbal reference of mine, is packed with anecdotal information and precise directions for making herbal remedies. It is also a strong reminder that, for centuries, women grew in their gardens simple herbs to help keep their families well. If the herbs you use to prepare your own remedies disappear from your healthfood store shelves, ask the owner if he/she has a petition you can sign to help protect these herbs from regulation. Or write to your local MP requesting that these beneficial, non-toxic herbs not be withheld from the consumer.

Chinese Bonjanmi Tea

This beverage is a mild diuretic and stomach soother and, according to the label, is guaranteed to make you beautiful. A green tea, Bonjanmi does not contain caffeine, and makes for a refreshing drink mid-afternoon.

James Barber's Ginger Tea

Put five cups of water in a pan, add a couple of inches of fresh, grated ginger root, half a lemon, a couple of cloves, and three tablespoons of honey or Sucanat. Simmer slowly, covered, for ten minutes. It is warming to the heart as well as the belly.

Calming Tea   I make this tea myself, using dried anise, chamomile flowers, ginger mint, penny royal (a herb to be used with great care and not to be taken by pregnant women), sweet cicely and vervain. Rub the dried herbs between the hands to make a manageable tealeaf size. I use this tea when I get cross and my body is over-tired. It usually restores my good humour and energy.

Cooking Herbs   In my herb garden, I grow Jerusalem artichokes, basil, chives, sweet cicely, chamomile, dill, ginger mint, lovage, lemon balm, marjoram, mint, oregano, parsley, penny royal, sage, sorrel, thyme, and vervain for soups, stews, sauces, and teas. From the beach, I gather kelp, dry it and grind it into powder to use as a salt substitute. In the fall, I make *bouquet garni* from all the herbs remaining in my garden. They are dried, ground, and given as Christmas gifts. The flavour varies from year to year, however my garden grows!

Oils

Omega oils   These oils are used as food supplements and are found in flaxseed, sesame, avocado, and almond oil. They are delicious when used in salad dressings, with rice vinegar and fresh herbs.

**Evening
Primrose oil** A rich source of essential fatty acids, and an antioxidant. It promotes healthy immune system function.

Cod liver oil Contains essential fatty acids that can lubricate and penetrate joints and muscles. I started taking two tablespoons of cod liver oil and two tablespoons of citrus juice two hours before breakfast. When I learned citrus fruits were not suitable for me, I changed to cod liver oil capsules.

Massage Oils

**Dandelion
oil** Provides deep penetration when massaging stiff necks, sore backs and arthritic knees.

**Rosemary
oil** Improves circulation, and aids mobility of stiff joints.

**St John's
Wort** Formerly called 'the blood of Christ' by medieval herbalists, because of its bright yellow flowers that turn oil a deep rich red, when steeped in it. This oil can be diluted with almond oil to be massaged into the skin where there is nerve injury. In times of stress, I put a few drops in my bath. Afterwards, I rub a little down my breastbone and across my solar plexus. Its familiar aroma gives me a sense of peace.

Mugwort oil   This oil is good for breaking up all forms of constriction, such as sore muscles, or bruises that tend to be blue in colour. It is beneficial to women during childbirth, and also for menstrual discomfort. A small amount in a bath is a helpful aid to sleep.

Marigold oil   Marigold is also known as Calendula. I love to make this oil myself. I have in my garden some Scotch marigolds in their umpteenth generation. I have transferred them to each new house we have moved to over the years. In the late summer, I gather the flower heads, and macerate the golden petals in almond oil. Placing the jar on a windowsill to be warmed by the sun, I tip and roll the jar periodically until I feel it is time (usually between 10 and 14 days) to pour the mixture through several layers of cheese cloth lining a kitchen sieve. When most of the oil has drained, I gather together the top of the gauze and squeeze out the last few drops, then bottle the beautiful golden liquid. I use this oil to soothe inflammation on or under the skin. It is an excellent first-aid remedy and a wonderful tummy rub used before childbirth to prevent stretch marks.

Other Natural Remedies

The well-known medical diagnostician and psychic healer, Edgar Cayce, prescribed countless natural therapies and remedies during his lifetime. Known as the 'sleeping prophet' because he appeared to sleep while receiving profound healing information for his clients, Cayce gave some

15,000 readings, all of which were documented. He died in January 1945, leaving behind a wealth of information.

With friends from the Association for Research and Enlightenment, I attended a seminar given by Edgar Cayce's son, Hugh Lynn Cayce. The Association continues to explore the work done by Edgar Cayce, and his son lectures on his father's works, giving us additional insights into the healing gifts of this incredibly unassuming man. It was at these seminars that I learned the practice of reverie.

For many years, I have used Cayce's recommendations for massage oils, various enemas, packs, and healing baths. However, I feel the following castor oil pack is one of Cayce's most powerful healing tools for chest congestion, strains and cysts. It is particularly good for drawing out toxins and inflammation from arthritic joints.

Supplies required:

wool flannel 10" wide by 10-12" long
1 diaper pin
1 tinfoil bread pan
4-6oz castor oil (oil of Palma Christi) soaked into the folded flannel
2 large towels
1 piece of plastic sheeting

Warm the oil-soaked flannel in a pan in the oven, being careful not to overheat it. Spread one towel on the bed, and lie down, applying the pack to the area of the body to be treated. Cover with the plastic sheeting. Wrap the second towel around this, fastening it securely with the diaper pin. Place heating pad on top of the towel to maintain the warmth of the pack. Rest for 1-1/2 hours. Take off the pack and return it to the tinfoil pan. Wrap in plastic and store for future use. Wash skin with baking soda in warm water.

It is desirable to do this for three consecutive nights, resting for one night and repeating again for three nights, if necessary. Each individual must use his/her own personal pack.

For further details of Edgar Cayce's drugless therapies, see Dr Harold Reilly's book listed in the Selected References and Further Reading at the end of the book.

Essential Oils

Valerie Ann Worwood's *Complete Book of Essential Oils and Aromatherapy*, and her companion book, *Fragrant Mind: Aromatherapy for Personality, Mind, Mood and Emotions*, are becoming widely used by therapists and those seeking natural healing approaches.

Essential oils are concentrated essences of flowers and fruit, herbs and plants. Aromatherapy is the preparation and application of these natural powerful medicines. Once used for centuries worldwide, they were put aside in favour of modern chemical drugs and imitation fragrances. These oils are now being rediscovered as safe, non-toxic healthcare aids.

During a 1998 seminar given by Valerie Worwood in Vancouver to introduce her new Mother Essences, she described these essences as vibrational and energetic dilutions of essential oils and water from the Chalice Well in Glastonbury, England. Water from this well is extremely pure as well as energetically potent. These essences can be used to support traditional aromatherapy treatment.

Three Australian Aromatherapists—Margaret Hall, Marilyn Harrison, and Bea Myers—who are also qualified Massage Therapists, have written a booklet, *Beyond the Basics of Aromatherapy*. It provides an easy-to-read, in-depth look at Aromatherapy for anyone wanting to enhance his or her own well-being.

Homeopathic Medicine and Bach Flower Remedies

Homeopathy is based on the Law of Similars, which states that the most effective medicine for an illness is one which could, in large doses, produce symptoms very much like those that are being treated. This principle has been known and used since ancient times but was first developed into a system by the great German physician, Samuel Hahnemann, at the end of the eighteenth century.

--The Homeopathic Home Care Kit: a User's Guide, by Neil Tessler, ND

Dr Edward Bach, a British physician who practised for many years as a Harley Street consultant and bacteriologist, gave up his position in 1930 in order to perfect a system of healing with homeopathic remedies. The remedies were made from refined and distilled essences of plants, suspended in purified water, and stabilized with a small amount of brandy. Today, the Bach Flower Remedies are widely used in Europe and North America to treat a variety of emotional conditions. They work with the most subtle energy, balancing and healing body, mind and spirit.

The story of Dr Bach's early years spent tramping and identifying plants in the Welsh countryside captured my imagination. I was already curious about healing with herbs and flowers because of the affinity I had with my own Welsh grandmother. When I first began to study Dr Bach's remedies at the Holistic Health Institute in Santa Cruz, California, I was given an assignment to prepare a remedy for myself. I felt confused and unable to get in touch with the feelings that would guide me to a choice. And I was rather skeptical about a few drops of a solution alleviating any problem I might have. Nonetheless, I decided to put the remedies to the test by working with my greatest fear—that of large aggressive dogs jumping up on me (which, incidentally, is exactly what happened to my mother just before I was born). I chose Mimulus, a remedy for known fears, and Walnut, a link breaker and a remedy for transition and change—as well as for the skepticism that was inhibiting my understanding.

During the following week, while walking along the beach, I felt something being pushed into my hand from behind. A large yellow Labrador was offering me a stick, urging me to throw it for him. Without thinking, I hurled the stick far out towards the sea. In just a minute or so, he had retrieved it and was racing back to me, panting excitedly. He dropped the stick at my feet and we continued playing until I had to go back to class. I cannot say it was a miracle cure and that the fear never returned, but in that brief incident, I did experience a release from the phobic fear that usually gripped me when I was around dogs. (When we went to live at Thistledown, a very friendly little yellow Labrador pup came to live with us. We called her Anna and she had the same grin as my friend on the beach. She became our official greeter for visitors, leading them to my studio as if to say, "Here she is."

I have since had many moving experiences as a result of both making and taking flower essence remedies. I am convinced that this simple but dynamic way of healing and balancing the body/mind has a very valuable part to play in holistic healing, as an adjunct to traditional medicine.

Sometime after I began using Bach Flower Remedies (among other remedies) in my practice, I had the good fortune to visit Dr Edward Bach's Healing Centre at Mount Vernon in Sotwell, England. After walking through Dr Bach's garden, I sat for a while in his simple consulting room, feeling deeply moved. I had no idea then what a large part these remedies would play years later in my own recovery from osteoarthritis.

When I first injured my wrist, I took Dr Bach's Rescue Remedy for the shock and fear. This First Aid remedy has the following five components to calm the feelings experienced as a result of injury: Cherry Plum for fear; Clematis for the dreaminess of shock; Impatiens for the irritability one feels after slipping or falling; Rock Rose for extreme fear or panic; and Star of Bethlehem for all kinds of shock and the after-effects of trauma. This remedy is the most readily available of all the Bach Flower Remedies and can be found in most well-stocked healthfood stores.

There are many wonderful stories about the recuperative powers of Rescue Remedy. In his book, *Handbook of Bach Flower Remedies*, Phillip M. Chancellor describes case histories relating to the thirty-eight flower remedies as well as Rescue Remedy. In the early days of my practice, I made the Rescue Remedy formula from the five separate components and gave it to family, friends and clients to use. (The remedy was not sold in healthfood stores then.) I received a great deal of positive feedback. A small girl who had been stung by a bee was shocked and angry that it had 'bitten' her when she was just holding it. After sipping the remedy, the tears stopped and the sting was removed. The next day, there was no swelling or soreness. Another client took the remedy before going to the dentist to help calm his nerves and relax him. He reported that it worked. And a young student, terrified of taking exams, sipped the remedy in some water and became calm and focussed enough to take her exams and do well.

I have my own stories about Rescue Remedy. Some years ago, on a hot summer day, Ross was working on our house at Thistledown. He was on the roof repairing a window frame when his support broke. He fell backwards, landing heavily on his heels, then falling flat on his back. He lay, winded, unable to move. The two young men working with him helped him into the house. As the story goes in our small community, these two men stopped to have a beer on their way home from work and regaled the people in the local pub with what had happened: "We helped this old guy into his house, his wife ran her hands all over him, put some drops into a small glass of water, and he sat there and sipped it. After lunch, he came back out to help us and spent the rest of the afternoon hauling sheets of Gyproc around. He seemed right as rain. Never seen anything like it!"

In the early stages of dealing with my arthritic condition, my lifestyle changes initially lessened my discomfort, but then, later, the discomfort accelerated, uncovering deep feelings of distress from past traumas that I did not initially recall. This pattern is described as 'peeling the onion.' As we release layer after layer of limiting experiences, we move towards an emotional balance within ourselves, and begin experiencing an accompanying improvement in all aspects of our being. While I worked on these emotions using other therapies, I continued using the gentle, non-invasive Bach remedies.

Although a scientist, Dr Bach considered intuition to be the deepest form of wisdom. Used in natural healing, it is an inherent skill available to us all.

In the foreword to *Handbook of the Bach Flower Remedies,* by Phillip M. Chancellor, Dr Bach is quoted as saying, "Let not the simplicity of this method deter you from its use, for you will find the further your researches advance, the greater you will realize the simplicity of all creation.

"Take no notice of the disease; think only of the outlook on life of the one in distress.

"Final and complete healing will come from within, from the Soul itself which, by this beneficence, radiates harmony throughout the personality when allowed to do so...the remedies cure, not by attacking the disease, but by flooding our bodies with the beautiful vibrations of our Higher Nature, in the presence of which disease melts away as snow in the sunshine. There is no true healing unless there is a change in outlook, peace of mind, and inner happiness."

When prescribing a homeopathic remedy for someone, the practitioner invites that person to describe how he or she is feeling. The practitioner listens carefully to the description of the symptoms or problems, and observes the individual's behaviour. Body language, signs of nervousness or low energy, twisting of hands or limbs, and avoidance of direct eye contact are some of the indicators the practitioner uses to make an appropriate choice.

When preparing a remedy, the practitioner enters into a contemplative state to access his or her source of innate wisdom. Using sterile conditions, the practitioner then blends pure spring water with a little brandy to stabilize it, and the chosen essences, in a small bottle. (The bottle usually has a glass dropper attached to its top, with a small rubber valve that enables the user to release a specific number of drops into the mouth under the tongue.) The contents of the bottle are then agitated by tapping the base of the bottle sharply against the heel of the hand. When giving dosage instructions, I include short notes on the healing properties contained within the flowers, herbs or sea life used. Lastly, a suitable affirmation may also be given to hold the individual's focus while the remedy is taken at regular intervals throughout the day. All essences contain their own unique signature that allows for specific natural healing to take place.

Muscle testing can also be used to help determine the most appropriate remedy. In this procedure, if the remedy is beneficial, the tested muscles remain strong. If it is of no benefit to the person being tested, the muscles grow weak and cannot stay locked. Using a pendulum, like dowsing for water, is another method of divination. When prescribing a flower essence remedy, I prefer to take the information I have gleaned in our consultation and then allow my intuitive sense to guide me in selecting the most appropriate combination. When I feel a need for clarity, I muscle-test as well.

One of the most highly regarded recent publications on the subject of energetic medicine (covering the fields of homeopathic remedies, flower essences, crystal healing, therapeutic touch, acupuncture, herbal medicine, and much more) is *Vibrational Medicine: the New Choices for Healing Ourselves*, by Richard Gerber, MD. On the cover, it states:

> *Doctors are beginning to reconceptualize human beings as more than just bodies of flesh and bones. They are beginning to understand that we possess unique energy systems that help to maintain health.*

Sea and Wildflower Essences

In the last twenty years, there have been other flower essences developed following Dr Bach's principles. Sabina Pettit and her company in Victoria, BC, for example, have developed a series of Sea Essences. As an acupuncturist, Pettit added another dimension to the generic remedy information by listing the chakra, meridian, key words and specific challenges that apply to the properties of each remedy, together with a short affirmation.

Here, on the West Coast, many of us walk along the seashore as we search for answers to difficult questions, or meditate to the sound of the timeless seas. It made sense to me that essences from the sea could benefit the people I worked with. As my clients and I used these twelve sea essences, we began opening up to deeper levels of awareness and understanding of the roles we could play in our own healing.

On one occasion, when I ordered some Sea Anemone essence from Sabina Pettit, I noticed that it came with new information that recommended stronger dosages of Pacific Sea Essences for use both sublingually and in the bath. I pondered this for a moment and got the feeling that I needed to take this particular remedy myself, at the increased dosage. The affirmation that came with this Sea Essence read: "For acceptance of self and others, by taking responsibility for one's own reality, allowing oneself to be organized by the Universe." Sabina Pettit subsequently told me that their most recent research with Anemone essence showed that it was most helpful for those suffering from osteoarthritis or other chronic pain.

Later, the Native Wildflower and Spring Flower series were developed by Pettit's company. In her book, *Energy Medicine*, Pettit tells a beautiful story about her work with both sea and flower essences and the guidance she received from the sea and nature spirits. More recent discoveries have since been made by her company through the use of gems and crystals.

The Flower Essence Society in Nevada City, USA, produces a wide range of flower essences and therapeutic oils which I have enjoyed using. In one of the society's newsletters, I noticed the following quote from Dr Edward Bach: "The need is NOW for those who have knowledge of Certain Herbs to go and teach all people how they may use them." The Society also describes its research program, and uses flower essences to help many small children suffering from physical or emotional traumas, learning disabilities, and other ailments that breed in the poverty-stricken and war-torn countries of the world.

Another remarkable figure in the field of flower essences is Machaelle Small Wright. Together with a group of dedicated people, she co-founded the Perelandra Centre for Nature Research in Virginia. In the spirit of the Findhorn gardens in Scotland, Machaelle has been working on and researching a natural garden. She works directly with nature's intelligences, known as Devas and spirits, in a co-creative relationship. Her book, *Behaving as if the God in all Life*

Mattered, describes her early experiences which propelled her to create the Perelandra garden.

Using Dr Bach's principles, the Perelandra company has produced a wide range of essences, most of which I have used. I am particularly grateful for the Rose II essences. This series carries elements that help balance the central nervous system, the body's sacrum at the base of the spine, the cranials (head bones), and the cerebrospinal fluid. These remedies are most efficacious for those experiencing an expanded state of being that challenges them physically, mentally or emotionally. They are designed to help individuals through different levels of the expansion experience, and have proved invaluable to me.

The Perelandra kinesiology technique (a form of muscle testing) is described by simple diagrammatic instructions contained in each series box of essences. I sometimes use it to check my own intuitive process when selecting flower essences or any other herbal, or aromatherapy substance.

Perelandra has a remedy series that addresses the stirrings of the soul that come into our consciousness when we are ready and able to listen to them. They also have a Viral, Bacterial and Fungal series that I find very effective.

Machaelle Small Wright makes available to us many of the Perelandra Papers which are translations of discussions and instructions she receives from nature's intelligences. Though not easy reading, they are intriguing and informative. The centre does not offer certification for flower essence practitioners, but teaches and encourages everyone to learn how to effectively use the essences for themselves and their families.

The most wonderful and amazing self-conducted meditative experience I learned from Machaelle is a physical and spiritual healing connection called a MAP session. This is a co-creative process, done in conjunction with nature, for physical, mental and emotional balancing. It is designed to facilitate our inner processes when we feel stuck or jammed. Using Wright's book, *MAP: the Co-Creative White Brotherhood Medical Assistance Program,* as a guide, individuals can open up other dimensions of their being and explore the realms of self-healing by working in harmony with the highest part of themselves. I find these practices extremely valuable, and consider them to have huge potential for healing in the next century.

Chapter 7 / Exercise: No Gain with Pain

To be what we are, to become what we are
capable of becoming, is the only aim in life.
—*Baruch Spinosa*

Self-Massage, Stretching and Breathing

Massage is invaluable for improving the circulation and flexibility of the body. It is also a gentle way to release the toxins held in the joints and muscles of arthritic limbs. From earliest times, this form of healing has been the most basic and essential way of nurturing ourselves and others.

Each morning, upon waking, I lie on my back and begin my first stretches by pushing my heels and legs down in the bed, stretching thigh and calf muscles and spreading my toes and rotating my ankles in both directions. Then I lie still, consciously relaxing my lower body. Next, I reach with my arms up towards the ceiling, inching up first the right hand and arm, then the left, so that I feel a gentle lift in the shoulders. I rotate my wrists as I did my feet, then lower my arms and hands to my chest, taking a deep breath and releasing it with a satisfying sigh from deep within my chest. Then I lie still for a moment, consciously relaxing feet, legs, torso, arms and hands.

I get up and go to the bathroom where I drink the first of my daily six glasses of room-temperature, pure spring water, and swallow one Devil's Claw root tablet. After a quick shower or bath, I return to sit on the side of my bed. While my body is still warm and moist, I begin to massage my limbs with almond oil and a few drops of St John's Wort oil.

With both hands, I hold the right foot and rub in between the toes, around the instep and arch, circling the ankles. I then make long strokes up the leg to encircle the knee. Using a slight kneading motion, I continue up the thighs and do a figure-eight circular movement over and around each hip and buttock, two or three times. I do the same on the other side, always moving towards the heart.

I then massage each finger within the loose clasp of the other hand, circling the wrist in the same way with the hand open, and fingers softly curling. I then use long strokes up to the elbow, encircling it, moving up and around the shoulder, gently pulling up, over and down the chest towards the heart. I repeat this two or three times and then do the same on the left side.

I lie down again with knees bent and rest for a moment. With my hand flat and soft, I massage my belly in a clockwise motion, repeating the pattern until I feel the abdominal muscles relaxing.

I rest for a few minutes before returning to sit on the side of the bed. Next, I begin to massage the outer ribcage with downward strokes, while stretching gently away from the side being rubbed. I repeat this several times on both sides.

Back in bed, I sit straight-backed and comfortable with pillows supporting the spine, my knees lying as open and flat as they wish to go. You may feel a little stiff, at first, but if you place supporting pillows under your knees, the muscles of the inner thighs and lower spine will gradually loosen and stretch. This softening is very beneficial and will help keep the hips open and mobile.

I use the flat of my hands to gently massage the sides of the neck vertebra, stroking from the muscles on top of each shoulder, up into the hairline, and down and out to the outside edge of the shoulder and upper arm in a slow rhythmic movement. Then I gently rub the outer shell of each ear between thumb and first finger, slowly pulling the ear lobe to open the ear.

My hands and wrists receive extra time now that they are warm and relaxed from this massage and have lost most of the hot, tight feeling in the fingers and thumbs. I hold the palms of my hands away, pushing forward with the heel of each hand to open them wide. I stop and let the fingers naturally curl into their palms, in a loose fist. I then turn them to face me, almost closed. Very, very slowly, I begin to open them like a flower unfolding in the sun. The palms are now warm in the centre, and thumb and fingers push and stretch, slowly opening each hand as far as it can go. I hold that position for the count of six, then gently release them to curl back slowly, like a flower closing. I hold them in my lap to rest, with my non-dominant hand cupping the other, and bless them for having worked so hard for me.

Lastly, after rapidly rubbing the palms of my hands together to produce a soothing warmth, I place my hands over my eyes. I look into the darkness, taking a deep breath and slowly releasing it with a sigh. Relaxed, with my hands resting in my lap, I stop and enjoy for a moment this lovely sense of self-nurturing.

I complete this massage and stretching time with alternate nostril breathing—or Pranayama, as it is called in Sanskrit—before continuing my daily regimen. One can sit in a chair, feet flat on the floor, but I prefer to sit in bed with knees open and the soles of the feet together. My back is supported and straight, with pillows under my right elbow and knees, if needed. When I am comfortable, I close my eyes, still my mind, then place my right thumb against my right nostril. My ring and small fingers are poised, ready, beside my left nostril, while my first and second fingers are held together in an upright position. I focus my attention on the breath.

The basic practice of Pranayama is as follows: gently close the right nostril with the right thumb, while the first and second fingers softly touch the space between the eyebrows. Start by releasing the breath from the left nostril, then the first inhalation is taken through this nostril with a gentle normal breath. When the intake of the breath is complete, close the left nostril with the ring and little fingers. Lift the thumb from the right nostril to release that breath. When released, inhale through the right nostril and continue breathing through alternate nostrils for five minutes. To keep your arm from getting tired, it helps to rest your right elbow against your body. When the breathing pattern is complete, lower the right arm and sit with the hands resting in the lap.

It is important to note that you begin the first breath of the exercise on the exhalation and finish on the inhalation. This is different from most Western breathing exercises, which begin by taking a deep breath in. In his wonderful book, *Perfect Health*, Deepak Chopra advises that, in Pranayama, you do not need to take deep breaths; just let the breathing come naturally, but a little slower and deeper than usual. If, at any time, you feel like breathing through the mouth, you can do so until you are ready to resume the exercise. Dr Chopra's books deal with many aspects of body/mind healing and have been a valuable source of information and inspiration for me.

Other Forms of Exercise

A variety of exercise forms is needed by those with osteoarthritis in order to find a balance of movements that do not cause too much fatigue yet keep the body flexible and mobile. The old adage, 'no pain, no gain,' is now known to be invalid. Any exercise should be practised solely for the benefit of the participant, who must take responsibility for working as hard and as long as is comfortable for him or her. This is the time to adopt 'tortoise wisdom' and become a winner, one slow step at a time.

Yoga

In the 1950s, I was introduced to the practice of Hatha yoga stretching exercises to enable me to experience natural childbirth. Ten years later, I studied yoga with the Indian teacher Dr Bina Nelson, among others, who taught the classical form of yoga. I found that the practice of deep yoga stretches, breathing, meditation, and simple fasting techniques gave me a calmness and inner balance that led to a deepening sense of my inner being. In time, I became a teacher. I taught the usual mixed classes, but particularly enjoyed my young mothers' class, with their babies being cared for in an adjoining room. It was quite a challenge for them to lie in the final relaxing pose at the end of the lesson, hearing their little ones getting restive nearby, and to gradually surrender themselves to having 'their time.' This, to me, is a most valuable practice for young mothers to learn—one that is ultimately of mutual benefit to mother and child.

Yoga can be practised at any age. From the elderly people in a seniors' home, to the energetic, rambunctious teenagers in our Alternative School program, I have seen every age and shape managing to stretch their tight limbs and 'let go.' With gentle practice, they can relax tense places in their bodies until they feel the answering wave of quiet energy and inner stillness.

Even with osteoarthritis, I still continued to practise simple yoga postures. My chiropractor suggested I take a class with a well-supervised group in order to expand my range of movement. I found such a group and began practising Iyengar Hatha yoga in a beginner's class. In previous years, I was wary of this more robust form of yoga, afraid of hurting myself.

However, in the fall of 1993, I began taking a class with an extremely well-trained Iyengar yoga instructor, Carol, who is also a massage therapist. With her eagle eye, she can spot an overextended limb or incorrectly positioned foot in a trice. Her assistant moves through the class, helping to make postural adjustments. Participants use canvas belts to help extend legs, foam blocks to cushion necks, and chairs to modify postures and support bodies.

During the class, I found that my body needed careful supervision to enable me to make a wider range of motion and to hold the pose just a little bit longer each time I attempted it. After these stretching exercises, I greatly enjoyed the overall sense of well-being that came during the relaxing and breathing period at the end of the evening. I would arrive home very tired, and often feeling as if I had been 'on the rack,' but I was also elated. I was no longer imprisoned in my painful body! A hot Epsom salts and bicarbonate of soda bath ensured that I had little stiffness the next day. When that series of classes ended, I returned for the next ten-week session and rediscovered parts of my body that were flexible and capable of being extended with little discomfort. I felt this was a re-surfacing of former flexibility from my past yoga experience to help my body regain some of its former strength. It is a bit like getting on a bicycle, after years of not riding, and finding that you have not forgotten how to ride.

I still attend fall, winter and spring classes of Iyengar yoga each year. This has enabled me to reframe my early-morning regimen to include more of the pre-class yoga stretches, and the standing and sitting poses I enjoy. My hands and wrists are considerably stronger now although, at times, I wear wristbands to support them in class.

Tai Chi

In the early years of my quest for health, I was fortunate enough to attend an introductory seminar to Tai Chi with Master Al Huang. His beautiful book, *Embrace Tiger, Return to Mountain*, shows the elegance of this art and the way he teaches his students how "to move with the wind and water."

On a beautiful spring morning, I attended one of his classes on a grass-covered playing field. We were invited to imagine we were lightly holding a large balloon. We practised making slow, precise hand and foot movements until break time, after which we were called together again by the sound of Master Al Huang's wooden flute. There was very little talking. I knew this slow, mindful practice would suit the contemplative side of my nature.

The old adage, "When the student is ready, the teacher will appear," proved true for me many times on my journey. Five years later, I found my Tai Chi teacher here, on the Sunshine Coast. Merrilee was devoted to her discipline and a patient instructor. Ross and I attended her classes for three or four years. As I had sensed on that first spring morning with Master Al Huang, Tai Chi became an integral part of my contemplative life.

In 1994, as my sense of balance and flexibility returned, I was fit enough to attend an intensive five-day Tai Chi Retreat on a secluded lake shore in the Kootenays, BC.

The days were rigorous and long, and our accommodation quite spartan, but the food was excellent. Delicious non-dairy and wheat-free meals were available for those who desired them—almost a third of the people there.

I attended a class given by a rather over-zealous instructor who kept a small group of us constantly repeating a turned-out knee position. In my own enthusiasm, I forgot the rule of exercise being solely for my benefit, and pushed myself to keep up. I later suffered a severely swollen knee and decided to avoid that particular teacher's classes for the rest of the retreat. I was approached, however, by a kind-looking man, an acupuncturist, who was also attending the retreat. He had noticed what had happened and offered to treat the knee. In a day or so, the swelling began to subside, and the end of the story is that he is now our family acupuncturist and friend.

NIA

In the spring of 1993, I felt strong and well enough to attempt a new form of non-impact aerobics called NIA. This wonderful blend of martial arts, dance and yoga-like movements is a mind/body cardiovascular program that lifts the spirits and blows away the cobwebs. Beautifully demonstrated by our instructor, these exercise sessions brought a great release from physical and emotional tension. I perspired a great deal and drank lots of water to expel toxins naturally from my body. A gentle wind-down with yoga breaths and relaxing postures completed each session. Three months later, I found my enthusiasm was greater than my stamina level and I had to stop for a while. I now take part in the NIA aqua class instructed by Trish at the local swimming pool. The buoyancy of the water reduces the impact on the joints without detracting from the grace and expressive movement of the form.

Walking

One of my favourite ways to exercise outdoors is to walk while breathing deeply to encourage the gentle loosening of painful joints. No matter what stage of osteoarthritis one is in, this gentle form of exercise is highly beneficial. A simple way of healing and nurturing yourself, walking acts as a warm-up exercise, a time for deep breathing, watching nature, greeting neighbours, and feeling a sense of belonging. It does not matter whether you walk fast or for miles every day. Walk whatever way you can. At one point, I was walking with a cane and could only walk for five or ten minutes at a time. Eventually, taking one step at a time, I was able to walk again without a cane.

One summer, I walked three times a week with a young friend who was healing from a back injury. We began by breathing and doing our loosening-up exercises on the grass verge at the side of the road before setting off. Gloria was gingerly putting one foot in front of the other while I was keeping an eye out for any over-friendly dogs that might bowl me over. At the end of each day's walk, we shared a flask of tea on the grass by the sea. By summer's end, having supported each other on passably brisk walks, we were both more limber. My lower back and hips were loose and flexible, my wrists, elbows and shoulders were relaxed and soft, and Gloria was able to walk comfortably again. It was a great way to share a healing journey.

Feldenkrais Method

Moshe Feldenkrais, DSc, 1904-1984, pioneered an amazing method for discovering more skilful, comfortable ways of moving and feeling, thinking and acting. His Feldenkrais lessons help to improve flexibility, posture, breathing, balance, and coordination. The student learns to work smarter instead of harder to ease stiffness and pain. This process is gentle, stimulating, challenging, and fun.

My message therapist, Hélène, invited a Feldenkrais practitioner to come to her office and introduce some of her clients to this most beneficial method of retraining damaged and stiff joints. He gave several weekend seminars that helped me to relax and open painful joints and limbs. This was done slowly and gently, making what appeared to be minuscule movements that helped me remove the fear-clenching habit that people with osteoarthritis often have. He recommended the book *Relaxercise* (written and clearly illustrated by D. and K. Zemach-Bersin and Mark Reese), which provided more opening and strengthening exercises for me to try when I felt ready to go further.

Chapter 8 / Alternative Therapies

You consist of the faith that is in you.
Whatever your faith is, you are.
--The Bhagavad Gita

Being a responsible participant is one of the most important aspects of any therapy one may choose to undergo. In my quest for health-enhancing options, I was not attempting to *live* with osteoarthritis, but rather to manage it and, ultimately, recover from it entirely. Osteoarthritis is a disease that has no direct or predictable route from onset to complete disability, manageability, or recovery. Stages of appearing to be free from it can be followed by what seem to be unexpected setbacks. I found that these were the times when I had the opportunity to experiences a deeper knowledge of myself.

Inevitably, as I changed, I looked for practitioners who could encompass and understand these changes, using the particular skills they offered. And I learned that moving on from one practitioner to another, when I knew I was ready for the next stage of healing, did not in any way negate the value of the relationship I had with the previous caregiver. It was simply a matter of honouring my own instinctive needs and persevering in finding ways to meet them.

Massage sessions were always an on-going part of my healing program, and still are. The therapies I describe from a client's viewpoint are those I sought out as I needed that particular form of healthcare.

Each journey of discovery and healing is as unique as the individual who embarks upon it.

Reflexology

Reflexology is the ancient art of stimulating reflex points in the feet, hands and ears, which correspond to the glands and organs in various parts of the body. By massaging these parts, circulation is improved, toxins are released and eliminated, and the body's flow of energy is stimulated so that healing can take place naturally.

I first became aware of reflexology in the early 1970s, when I found a practitioner I went to monthly for nearly a year. Though many of her clients were skeptical about her practice, she spent the last three years of her life quietly introducing them to the benefits of this very effective approach to health. I eventually decided to train in reflexology myself.

Mrs K. McKenzie of Vancouver, BC, was another early reflexology teacher who operated despite the risk of being involved in what was then considered an 'illegal practice.' Now, thankfully, reflexology is widely practised and its many health benefits acknowledged by many members of the medical profession.

Reflexology is one of the least intimidating of all the bodywork therapies and a good place to start exploring them. In the reflexologist's workroom there is usually a diagram chart showing the reflex points on the feet and the corresponding body parts affected. Clients sit with legs extended towards the practitioner, and each foot is wrapped in a warm towel. The practitioner then works on one foot at a time, massaging various points to stimulate or release the respective organs and glands. The feet are like a map of the body, closely mirroring human anatomy. For example, the big toe refers to the head and eyes, while the base of that toe corresponds to the neck at the seventh cervical vertebra point—a spot in the body where a great deal of tension is often held. Working just below the small toe on the outside of the sole of the foot can greatly relieve tense or tight shoulders. The inside of each foot, from toe to heel, carries the reflexes for all the spinal vertebrae, and the lower portion of the foot, where the heel starts, is where the knee and hip points are found.

Congested spots explored by the practitioner are often painful, and the client is asked to breathe slowly and deeply until the discomfort subsides. It is usually followed by a sense of relief. Towards the end of the session, the crease between the base of the big toe and the second toe on the top of the foot is massaged to release the toxins loosened by the massage. Finally, the practitioner usually applies some warm essential oils, gently manipulating the loosened toe and foot joints into letting go of all residual tension. The feet are then wrapped in a towel, and the client is given a large glass of water to drink, to help flush the released toxins from the body.

Massage

Massage is the oldest, most natural way for human beings to express their affection for each other in a physical way. The core benefit of the massage is its unique ability to communicate without words. When carried out by a skilled practitioner, it can be a profoundly relaxing and therapeutic experience. The client lies on a massage table, draped with sheets that allow for the back, arms, legs and front of the body to be uncovered as each part is being worked on. Lying in this secure, cocooned way allows the individual to drift into a mentally and physically relaxed state. The depth of this self-awareness can be enhanced by the smell of herbs or floral essences that can be added to the massage oil.

The various techniques employed by a sensitive masseuse/masseur help reduce tension and anxiety. Having a massage can also represent a precious gift of time to oneself. Emotional pain long held in neck, shoulders, buttocks, belly, and leg muscles can surface and be released. Rhythmic breathing patterns demonstrated by the practitioner can offer another way for the person to participate and aid in their own private process.

As a medical health insurance client, I found that my one-hour sessions ended somewhat abruptly, leaving me little time to assimilate the process before leaving the room. However, there are many well-trained massage practitioners who give full-body massages that do allow sufficient time for their clients to assimilate any emotional and spiritual insights that may have occurred during the session. Finding the right practitioner to meet one's particular emotional, as well as physical, needs is therefore important.

After I stopped working in 1987, a young woman approached me, asking me to teach her the holistic elements of my work. Shelley already had a natural ability and sensitive nature. At that time, my body could only tolerate the most delicate and intuitive touch. She soon gave me massage sessions that reflected back to me her skill and sensitive awareness of my needs. We became good friends and, in due time, I became the godmother to her firstborn son.

In 1990, Hélène became my massage therapist. I made regular visits every month or so over the following five years. In 1993, when I discovered I had further degeneration of neck and lumber vertebrae, she was with me as I expressed my frustration or collapsed on her table just wanting release from my discomfort. After an hour in her quiet room, and in her gentle presence, I could go back out into my world feeling relaxed and nurtured.

Now I am happy to say that my hands and wrists have grown strong and comfortable enough for Shelley and me to exchange massages—although my contribution is a lighter and shorter version of my previous work. I enjoy our sharing—an opportunity to experience that place of deep concentration with another, and to feel the rhythmic movements of my flexible body as we breathe and release together. It reminds me just how far I have come on this journey, and that gives me a sense of peace and gratitude.

Under the umbrella term of massage lie many different schools of expertise. Swedish and Esalen techniques, for example, offer a variety of gentle ways to access stressful parts of the body. Polarity is a more subtle technique whereby blocked energy within the musculo-skeletal framework of the body can be released. The practitioner places his/her hands in prescribed positions until the release and balance of energy are achieved. Shiatsu is a more physical form of massage where pressure is applied along the body's meridians—the lines of energy that run from the head down the trunk, legs, and feet, and down the arms to wrists and fingertips. The nervous and immune systems are also stimulated. These practices promote the elimination of toxins and improve circulation, as does Jin Shin Do/Acupressure, a Japanese form of massage that breaks up deeply held tension or energy blocks and stimulates the flow of vital life energy.

Craniosacral Balancing

This form of bodywork involves a very subtle manipulation of the skull to stimulate the circulation of the cerebrospinal fluid around the brain. This, in turn, helps bones to resume their natural position, with the fluid acting as a lubricant and shock absorber for the brain. My practitioner Usha's skilful, sensitive touch loosened the constricted connective tissue around my neck vertebrae and head bones, bringing great relief. This physical release was often accompanied by an emotional one.

Reiki

Reiki (pronounced *ray-key*) is a Japanese word meaning 'universal life energy.' Practitioners of this form of bodywork radiate this healing energy through their hands, affecting the physical, emotional and mental levels of the client. The individual, clothed in loose garments and lying on a massage table, will feel the gentle touch and subsequent warmth of the practitioner's hands moving over his/her body. When the energy is brought to the focused and conscious awareness of the client, Reiki increases the body's natural ability to heal physical ailments. While relaxing in this safe and caring environment, clients may receive insights from within as to the cause of their disease or distress.

Therapeutic Touch

Therapeutic Touch is an energy transfer and balancing therapy first described in the early 70s by Delores Kreiger, a professor of nursing, and Dora van Gelder Kunz. It is a conscious and active healing process based on ancient healing practices. As the recipient lies comfortably, wearing loose clothing, the practitioner's intent is to help reduce stress and pain, while accelerating the healing process. Because the human energy field extends beyond the physical form, the Therapeutic Touch practitioner works four-to-six inches above the body, using the hands to balance the individual's energies.

Trager Therapy

Trager Therapy, developed by Milton Trager, MD, is another soothing form of bodywork, performed on a table. Wearing loose garments, the client experiences gentle, rhythmic rocking movements designed to profoundly relax, reassure, and comfort. The body, slowly and without mental effort, responds and begins to release old holding patterns in limbs, torso and spine. As the peaceful rocking continues, the individual often experiences relief from pain and a lovely sense of the body lengthening and expanding with ease.

Chiropractic Medicine

Chiropractic is the treatment of illness by physical manipulation, with the emphasis on the structural and neurological aspects of the body. Many of us have experienced this widely acclaimed healing art when a stiff neck is magically released with manipulation, and we feel the extraordinary relief that follows. Regular adjustments, manipulations and massage of chronically tight muscles help release pain from the pressure of movement in the skeletal structure. Those with arthritis tend to hold themselves in such a way as to 'favour' a limb to stop it hurting. This, in turn, puts pressure on other parts of the body, often resulting in misalignment.

In 1990, I began to receive treatments from a deceptively petite doctor of chiropractic, Christine Bird. At that time, I could not carry hot cooking pots from stove to sink in safety, and experienced a great deal of pain in my wrists, elbows and shoulders. I had experienced chiropractic adjustments before, but was fearful of the quick, strong movements made by some chiropractors. To begin the session, Dr Bird asked me to step onto a foot stand with a taut string attached to it. The heels of my feet were fitted into the base of this apparatus and the string was allowed to hang down my back, from my head to my toes. This simple device enabled Dr Bird to check my body alignment before beginning treatment. She also used kinesiology (muscle-testing) techniques before determining what the treatment should entail.

This form of chiropractic treatment enabled me to cope with the discomfort of osteoarthritis and keep me moving as naturally as possible. It also gave me constant reassurance that I could get stronger. Three years later, with my health improved, I went on holiday to Guatemala, confident that I could handle this rather active trip. I practised my daily exercise, breathing, and meditation regimen every morning without fail.

I did, however, fall down a gravelly bank, which resulted, a month later, in excruciating pain. X-rays showed damage to three cervical vertebrae. A month later, my knee gave way, and I needed a cane when going for short walks. More X-rays revealed damage to the lumbar spine. I took copies of my X-rays to Dr Bird, who examined them carefully. She looked thoughtful as I sat glumly waiting to hear for her prognosis.

"Well," she said, "I think you are going to be alright."

We began a week of intensive treatments and Dr Bird suggested I take the anti-inflammatory medication prescribed by my doctor while the vertebrae were slowly being adjusted.

Months of treatment ensued, and I did not appear to be responding in my usual way. Dr Bird suggested I go to a naturopathic physician for Vega testing to determine if I was eating incorrect foods for this osteoarthritic condition. Toxic foods as well as insufficient deep stretching exercises could be contributing to my loss of muscle strength.

The Vega test did show I was eating foods that I was allergic to, and this was remedied. I also found a yoga class that strengthened my body, increased my mobility and flexibility, and gave me great enjoyment.

I still go to Dr Bird for a check-up at regular intervals and am most grateful for her wise advice and constant care that helped me regain my health. However, when increased knee, low back and hip pain prevented me from getting out of the bath one day, I decided to move on to a highly regarded chiropractic doctor who practised Upper Cervical Chiropractic.

First he took three X-rays and analyzed them to determine a course of treatment. During the next three visits, after correction had taken place, my head and neck were restored to normal alignment, relieving the knee, low back and hip pain. The Upper Cervical Spine Adjustment taps into the body's innate intelligence, prompting it to return to a normal head and neck posture. I now require only an occasional adjustment.

Naturopathic Medicine

An important turning point in my healing journey was when I consulted Dr David Bayley, a naturopathic physician, to learn more about Vega testing, and what it could do to help me deal with osteoarthritis. I was immediately struck by his own obvious good health and his keen interest in helping me regain mine. He suggested doing a Vega test to determine which foods where unsuitable for me.

A Vega test uses an electronic acupressure instrument that is placed on various pressure points in the fingers. The device measures the body's electrical response to various substances, giving a negative or positive reading. By this means, it is possible to determine specific information about the patient's health. The process is painless. The patient sits in a chair holding a neutral electrode while the operator touches an acupuncture point on the tip of one of the patient's fingers. The operator then selects various ampoules containing different food substances and places them in the circuit. After each testing session, Dr Bayley would discuss the results and make suggestions or answer questions regarding my progress. Within four months, he had identified and helped me manage the food allergies that aggravated my osteoarthritic condition.

The information I have gleaned, together with a correct food plan for my particular needs, is probably the most valuable tool I have for maintaining my present state of vibrant good health.

Acupuncture

Health is a state of total harmony between the physical, emotional and spiritual elements of our being. A healthy person's *Qi* (the body's vital energy) moves smoothly, but when this energy is blocked, illness occurs. Acupuncture is the ancient Chinese healing art of using fine needles to stimulate invisible lines of energy running beneath the surface of the skin. This effects change in the body's energy systems, stimulating further healing. Acupuncture is good for a variety of conditions, including chronic, acute or painful disorders, infections, internal/external diseases, and cardiovascular, respiratory, and gastrointestinal problems, among others.

I was first introduced to the concept of holistic healing by Dr Harold Saita, a Japanese acupuncturist practising in West Vancouver, BC, in the 1960s. In those days, acupuncture was considered very exotic and strange. However, I was seeking relief from migraine headaches, and had heard of Dr Saita and his ancient healing art.

Sitting in the doctor's waiting room, I noticed a small, simply framed statement hanging on the wall. It said, *"It is God who doeth the work."*

I was requested to change into a paper gown and put paper slippers on my feet. In Dr Saita's healing room, we bowed to each other and spoke little. Instinctively I trusted this gentle man. Within three months, the migraine headaches from which I had suffered for sixteen years had been eliminated. And a spinal weakness, due to a severe teenage illness, was also alleviated by regular acupuncture sessions.

Of the many practitioners I consulted, Dr Saita was the first to stress the importance of holistic healing. He explained why, as humans made up of myriad systems, we cannot function effectively unless all these systems work together in harmony and balance. He was quite elderly when he retired in the 1970s, and was greatly missed by those who knew him. Up until shortly before his death, he devoted himself to teaching Western doctors the principles of the ancient healing art he practised with such dedication and elegance.

In the spring of 1994, I was referred to another Vancouver-based Chinese acupuncturist whose youthful face belied his years of experience. He placed needles with a delicacy I had not experienced since my time with Dr Saita, thirty years previously, and, as with Dr Saita, this acupuncturist spoke little. During each session, after being covered with a light blanket, I would fall asleep. Yes, with needles in my feet, hands, ears and neck, I would fall into a deep, deep sleep. I often slept for an hour or more. After the treatment, my energy became more balanced, bringing some relief from a pulsing beat around my left ear and jaw. However, unable to travel to Vancouver for a while, I decided to consult a local acupuncturist, Réjèan Roy, who lived on the Sunshine Coast.

When I arrived at his office, he took a detailed account of my history of osteoarthritis. His insightful questions gave me an opportunity to express my own feelings of why this pulsing sound persisted. Our first session brought relief both emotionally and physically. By the third session, the pulsing (due to energy congestion behind the ear, jaw and neck, possibly due to pressure from damaged neck vertebra) was gradually clearing. As I lay on the table during my last session, I looked up through the glassed-in roof, watching the clouds scudding through the sky, and had a sense that I really was on the last leg of this journey.

114

Ayurveda

Ayurveda, which means '*the science of life*,' has its roots in ancient Indian Vedic civilization. It uses a unique combination of exotic tropical herbs, blended according to Vedic science. This ancient tradition also deals with the aspects of social, ethical, intellectual and spiritual life, in order to bring about a state of perfect health. My interest was captured from early readings of the principles of Ayurveda when I learned that it recognized three different constitutions, or *doshas*—Vata, Kapha and Pitta. Most individuals are primarily one of these types, which is often combined with a few characteristics from one of the other *doshas*. Each constitution (or personality type) thrives on different foods, forms of exercise, and emotional environments.

In his best-selling book, *Perfect Health*, Dr Deepak Chopra explains how the Ayurvedic approach of selecting the correct foods, exercise, bodywork, and meditation for our particular body type can bring us to a balanced, healthy, and continually evolving way of life. I consulted an Ayurvedic physician and learned that I was of a Vata *dosha*, with some Pitta. With this information, the *Ayurvedic Cookbook* by Amadea Morningstar, with Urmila Desai, was of great help to me as I searched for new ways of preparing appropriate foods for my type.

In Dr Vasant Lad's book, *Ayurveda: the Science of Self-Healing, a Practical Guide*, I also found simple diagrams used in diagnosis as part of this ancient, sacred, holistic form of healing.

Kinesiology

Applied kinesiology is the science of biofeedback, through muscle testing, which identifies and corrects blockages in the body's energy and structural systems.

Intrigued by the concept, I decided to take a three-day Educational Kinesiology course called Brain Gym I, a delightful and informative introduction to the study of balancing and enhancing whole brain learning. To quote Garry Gallagher, the bio-kinesiologist who taught this course, "Brain Gyms are exercises for releasing physical, mental and emotional blocks to learning. This promotes advanced body/mind integration that helps us to achieve our dreams, increase overall good health and cultivate happiness." (The course material was taken from the Brain Gym Handbook by Paul E. Dennison, PhD, and Gail Dennison.)

Before beginning our exercises, we were instructed to drink a glass of water. This was to ensure good electrical conductivity, as the muscle-testing process relies on the body's electrical currents to pass messages between the brain and sensory organs.

The following are examples of exercises that can be done anywhere, at any time, to bring the brain back into balance.

The 'Cook's Hook-Up' involves crossing the ankles, first left over right, and then right over left. Cross the arms at the wrist, with palms facing each other, and then clasp the fingers together. Allow the crossed hands to rest in the lap. I find this a great way to become centred and relaxed at any time during the day or night.

'Lazy Eights' is an exercise that enhances concentration and focuses both hemispheres of the brain on the task at hand. It is achieved by making horizontal figure-eight shapes in front of your line of vision, using an upraised thumb. Extend the arm, loosely clench the fist, and use the upraised thumb as a pointer for the eyes to focus on. Do not move the head as you make the figure eight.

'Cross Crawl' involves standing with bent elbows moving rhythmically and diagonally across the body as the opposing knee is raised in a stepping motion to meet it. This exercise creates a sense of balance within, and increased coordination between, the two sides of the brain and the body. It is also a very natural instinctive movement for babies to make while lying in their cribs on their backs, crooning and kicking like the wise little beings they are.

These brain-integration exercises are now commonly described in educational journals, and many teachers are interested in bringing Brain Gym to schoolchildren. Some teachers already use these exercises to centre and relax their students, while also bringing a sense of fun and unity into the classroom.

Chapter 9 / Dealing with Emotions

Don't exclude yourself from precious moments,
warm encounters, beautiful attitudes, majestic discoveries,
flowing intimacies, sensory developments, for these are
the jewels in the crown of your destiny.

--Waltern Rinder

By the summer of 1991, I was making steady physical progress. Random patterns of pain occurred less often, and I was experiencing new and exciting shifts within myself. However, at the first sign of a setback, I would experience panic and anger. Just thinking about the likelihood of osteoarthritis rendering me helpless or dependent would make me flush all over with a painful heat. It was not like the heat of inflamed muscles or joints, but rather a flushing that seemed to come from somewhere deep inside my body.

I discovered that my massage therapist, Carol, was also a certified practitioner of the Rosen Method—a form of bodywork that allows unexplored, deeply buried emotions to come into consciousness. Intuitively, I felt that this approach might help me, and decided to book a session.

In retrospect, I believe my intuitive self was waiting for the right time, place and person to come together so that I could begin the delicate process of emotional release.

I was to discover that my feelings of panic and anger were rooted in deeply buried memories. There were violent times in my young life. With the empathetic support and skill that Carol offered, it became possible for me to re-live these memories of fear and abandonment, and to verbalize them. As

I looked at these situations from my adult perspective, the feelings of helplessness and immobilization began to shift. I was no longer a vulnerable child. I was now following a positive course for healing the body, mind, spirit and emotional aspects of my whole being.

A Rosen Method session is designed to enable the client to get deeply in touch with him/herself. You are asked to lie on a table on your stomach. The practitioner massages the tight muscles with just the right amount of pressure to make it possible to feel that part of your body from the inside, while you breathe into those places, helping to bring repressed feelings to the surface.

Open dialogue with the Rosen Method practitioner is vital in establishing a mutual trust so that the forgotten deep feelings and old memories have a safe space in which to emerge. This rediscovery and reconnection of very intimate parts of oneself nurtures the heart and soul back to wholeness.

This work facilitates personal transformation. We are often aware of certain self-limiting patterns within ourselves and, through releasing old conditioning and emotional barriers, we can regain our authentic selves.

When working as a holistic practitioner, I found that clients' long-buried childhood memories, scenes and emotions surfaced when deep muscle releases were achieved through bodywork. And, in my studies of Transactional Analysis, which examines the principles of parent, adult and child ego states, I discovered that there was a language that helped us communicate with and understand these emotional expressions. Hence, I came to believe that there is more than one inner child. If you close your eyes for a moment and call up images of yourself as a child, you will probably see several pictures of yourself at different ages, in particular circumstances that you remember quite clearly. I feel it is the smallest and, probably, the most frightened of those children who wait until we are really strong before they can come forward to tell their stories. Through the Rosen Method, I had found this 'small one' who had, up to then, been unable to express how sad, angry and frightened she had been. The next step was to use this information and work with it. There is not always sufficient time to do so in a one-hour Rosen session, but further work can be done by the individual, using this information.

Marion Rosen, the founder of the Rosen Method, summed up her therapy well when she said: "This work is about transformation from the person we think we are to the person we really are. In the end, we cannot be anyone else."

Rebirthing

Rebirthing, also known as conscious breathing (or vivation), is a therapy developed by Leonard Orr and Sondra Ray. This special breathing technique is designed to activate memories, images or emotions locked into the body's cellular memory.

The therapist guides the client through a circular breathing pattern to help him/her re-experience any deeply buried physical or emotional feelings that have caused psychological blocks to health.

The practitioner provides a totally private and safe environment for the client who lies comfortably covered on a low bed or table. The session begins with an introduction to the rebirthing breath—an accentuated inhalation, immediately followed by a completely relaxed exhalation. As this rhythm is established between practitioner and client, muscles begin to relax, and sometimes a buzzing sensation is felt in parts of the body, indicating that the deepening process has started. The client may describe any images and feelings that surface, and this feedback is used by the Rebirther to facilitate the session.

In the weeks that followed my Rosen Method sessions, I began to actively experience feelings of outrage. When they welled up, I expressed them privately through tears and pillow-thumpings that released this pent-up energy. Gradually, new feelings emerged, and they were like coloured beads of new understandings, strung together, that I could hold and feel. This inner integration was made up of fragments of memories and feelings that all belonged to me, and I knew them. I was 'claiming' all of me!

When I was ready to release all the images and feelings that no longer benefited me, another woman was waiting to help me on this journey. This one, a most gifted and compassionate Rebirthing therapist, was my daughter, Mahara. We laughingly say that we have been together in different roles with each other for many lifetimes. This time, I happen to be Mahara's mother, but we are both each other's teacher.

I had had several rebirthing sessions with Mahara over the twenty years she had been practising, and often wanted to turn back from a place of dread that I could not enter. Mahara, in her wisdom, had respected this boundary that I was not yet ready to cross. Now, through the Rosen Method, I had discovered what the dread was. I was willing to move on again, knowing my little kid was safe with me. As my child within relived those once-deeply-buried experiences, the strong, loving young woman guiding me was my own physical child, Mahara.

We worked in my room by the sea, in an atmosphere of timeless, limitless space. As we breathed together, I journeyed within to a place where my own powerful and strongly nurturing woman could come forward and speak aloud to the people who had harmed me—knowingly or not. When I felt ready, those old feelings were offered up to be forgiven and transmuted by the light. My gratitude for the love and trust Mahara and I share brought me to a place of peace and reaffirmation of my life.

Opening wounded parts of ourselves is clearly designed to integrate and accept all aspects of the self. This is why I feel that forgiving ourselves and others is an essential part of this work. Usually, early trauma prompts us to find different ways of dealing with similar difficult situations we encounter in adult life, to avoid being hurt again, but this is still a reaction to the past. Doing this work gives individuals the freedom to act in a healthy, non-reactive, balanced way.

I believe we do need to reach back to that inner child and to envelope it with the necessary acts of caring, known only to ourselves, that the child needs in order to heal those hurts. The young, bud-like aspects of ourselves that got squashed by fear can bloom again in our adult lives in quite astonishing ways. Each time we heal a part of ourselves, we come closer to embracing the unique, multi-faceted beings we were born to be.

Dharma Path

The Dharma Path is the path of service we choose to follow at a spiritual, soul level. In his book, *The Path to Love*, Deepak Chopra, MD, says, "Choosing your own dharma determines completely how happy, successful, and loving you will be in your lifetime."

I have followed the path of a healer, with my own healing journey bringing to me people who faced serious health challenges. Many of these had a terminal illness that created within them the desire to find a conscious sense of inner healing and the innate sense of the goodness of life. This alone made it possible for them to embrace the next stage of their journey.

From 1992 to 1995, I worked with five men and women who were dealing with crisis situations or terminal illness in their lives. It was a salutary experience for me, sharing with them their anguish and courage as they moved through these difficult challenges in their lives. One couple carried an aura of acceptance and peace right up to the time they died. Louise had made a great contribution in bringing classical music concerts here to the Coast. She was asked by a friend what she would like to have sung at her funeral service. She replied, "I would rather hear you sing while I am still alive." Recognition of her request spread throughout the community. Time was growing short but, in two weeks, choirs, solo singers, and instrumentalists were ready. Flowers and food to be shared afterwards were brought by many. The local arts centre was packed with people who had come to give their gift of music to Louise. With amazing grace and strength, she and her family sat and received all the love and admiration each person could pour from within. They performed for her, her family, and all of us who were close to her. We were a community inspired. The atmosphere was charged with life, and it was her *life,* not her death, that we were celebrating. Her death came quietly about three weeks later.

On that special day, I watched a close friend of Louise, who was also dying, play a favourite piece for her on his guitar. He lifted his head from the instrument and looked into her face. Like him, I knew that the gift we gave of ourselves became our own healing.

Chapter 10 / Meditation and Visualization

Work in the invisible world
at least as hard as you do in the visible.
—Jalal-ud-Din Rumi

The following self-healing practices proved very useful to me during my healing journey.

Colour Therapy

Colour Therapy was used in ancient times in the temples of light and colour in Egypt, as well as in early Greece, China and India. I was first introduced to this form of therapy through the documented research of Edwin Babbitt and Dinshah Ghadial, pioneers in colour therapy literature.

I use colour to enhance the therapeutic properties of water. I fill a glass jug with fresh spring water, wrap it in coloured plastic filter sheets, and place it in direct sunlight. The pranic forces of the sunlight charge the water with the energetic frequency of the particular colour filter used. The water is then drunk as a remedy. (These filters can be obtained from the College of Psycho-Therapeutics, White Lodge, Kent, UK.)

There are seven major energy centres—called chakras—running from the tailbone to the top of the head. These centres resonate with colour, and have specific functions and properties. The first (or root) chakra, located in the tailbone area, is red—the colour with the lowest frequency energy—and has to do with survival and being grounded in the earth. The second chakra, located in the lower abdomen, is orange; this is the spleen/sacral chakra, relating to sensual emotion and creativity. The third chakra is located at the solar plexus, and its yellow energy has an effect on our intellectual nature. These first three chakras make up the triad of grounding functions. The fifth, sixth and seventh chakras are considered to represent the spiritual triad—the gateway to the spiritual nature of the higher mind—with the fourth chakra acting as the bridge between both triads. This chakra, located at the heart, is green and has the vibration of harmony and balance. The throat chakra (the fifth energy centre) vibrates to the colour blue and has to do with verbal communication. The third eye (the spot between the eyebrows) is the location of the sixth chakra, which is indigo; focussing on this colour and centre helps us to achieve clarity and depth when meditating. The seventh, or crown, chakra, at the top of the skull, is violet-magenta in colour and is considered to be the highest vibrational centre associated with deep inner searching, which allows us to enter into higher states of consciousness.

Leonardo da Vinci maintained that, "The power of meditation could be enhanced tenfold if carried out under the influence of violet rays passing through stained-glass windows of a quiet church."

Headache sufferers can often benefit from sitting in front of a sunlit window, with a piece of violet stained glass fastened to it so that the violet light is focused on their head.

Imagining colour within various parts of the body while meditating can be a healing experience. As I sit quietly after my morning exercises, I imagine myself wrapped in series of colours. I begin with violet, which is thought to help purify the body and mind. Then I visualize rich emerald green surrounding my energy field, and begin to feel my emotional body being harmonized and balanced. I picture a cloud of sapphire or gentian-blue floating over me, and direct the energy of this colour to regenerate and rejuvenate my entire physical structure. A deep-to-lemon-coloured yellow stimulates the mental processes and activates creativity. A morning mist of pink evokes a sense of peace, whereas a cloak of magenta moves me to a place of inner compassion for myself and others. I slowly return to my surroundings, opening my eyes, feeling refreshed in body, mind and spirit.

Meditation

Always meditate on your own inner self.
—Baba Muktananda.

Meditation has many health benefits. It reduces heart rate and blood pressure, soothes the mind, relaxes the physical body, reduces stress, and provides access to our inner wisdom, among other things.

I look forward to spending time in my inner world. It is not always easy to stop the mind-chatter, but I sit and focus on the breath gently coming in and out of my body. Sometimes I manage to reach a moment of absolute stillness in which I hear nothing but my breathing.

Meditation is essentially a contemplative way of communing with the self. To do this, sit comfortably on the floor. Make sure you are unlikely to be interrupted. Sit, aided by pillows, or in an armchair so that your back and arms are supported and your feet are placed flat on the floor. Place a shawl or scarf around your shoulders to keep you warm, close your eyes, and begin slow, deep breathing.

I use a wooden *sieza* bench, designed for meditation. It is about eighteen inches wide and six-to-eight inches high, with a sloping seat. When I kneel with my legs and feet behind me along the floor, I slide the bench under my bottom as I take a sitting position. The bench slopes forwards so that my tailbone is raised. This position helps to take a great deal of weight off tender or stiff muscles and joints, while allowing the back to assume a relaxed but upright posture. I relax my hands, palms up, in my lap, with my dominant hand cradled by the other.

Meditating in nature can be very therapeutic for ruffled emotions or an overly active mind. Leaning against a tree, absorbing its strong, solid stillness, is very grounding. In my garden, I practise a walking meditation. With eyes half-closed, looking through my lashes, this soft focus draws me towards the shimmering colours of the flowers. I centre on one and allow my gaze to explore the shape and texture, the shadows and light. I become conscious of its fragrance and seem to merge into the very centre of it. As the minutes pass in this simple magical world of nature, I am momentarily released from my daily round.

In his book, *Vibrational Medicine*, Dr Richard Gerber writes extensively and scientifically on alternative methods of diagnosis and healing. He also talks of passive and active ways of meditating, stressing the importance of activating and cleansing blockages of the chakras (the body's seven major energy centres described above). Since each of these centres is connected to a major nerve plexus and gland, cleansing and unblocking them can bring relief to the corresponding gland, while reducing the emotional blockage occurring within the personality, which indirectly causes organ dysfunction in the body. The various flower essences, crystal and colour therapies work at the level of the chakras to assist in energy balancing. Chakras can also be cleansed and balanced through yoga, whereby specific postures and sounds are used to activate each energy centre.

Meditating to music can soothe, relax and energize. I use music to change my energy when I feel 'stuck.' By moving my body with the music, I can move the energy. Music—from plain song to the richness and vastness of what we call our classical form—has been used for centuries as a way of transcending our earthly limitations. Composers such as Bach, Beethoven, Mozart, Mendelssohn, Scriabin,

Schubert and Wagner were aware that meditation opened them to their heights of creativity.

Meditating to the music of ancient cultures, with their primal rhythms and sounds from drums, strings, and wind instruments, often promotes a response in our bodies as our minds are lulled by the music.

When meditating to music, I move with my eyes in soft-focus, allowing the sounds and vibrations to lead me into forgetting my physical limitations and allowing the sound to dance through me.

Chanting

Chanting is an ancient practice that uses our vocal chords as an instrument for sound that can calm or invigorate us. It allows me to express, in a mindful way, energies held in feelings I am not always aware of. As I chant the sacred phrase, "Om Namah Shivaya" (I honour the God within), the rest of my body softens and gently moves to the rhythm, and I become the sound. Chanting often brings moments of self-revelation. It is a way of opening us up to the wisdom within.

Affirmations and Visualizations

Affirmations and visualizations are both ways of communicating with the self, using the mind's eye, for the purpose of retraining ourselves in positive ways. Through this process, we can let go of old conditioning, and old habits of thought or speech, which hold us back from finding satisfaction within our lives. An affirmation is a phrase of positive intention written or spoken repetitively. For example, statements such as "I am willing to receive..." or "I deserve to receive..." can be used to help create what you want in your life. Sometimes these repeated phrases elicit an underlying feeling, contrary to what is being expressed. Exploring the thoughts and feelings that contradict our expressed desires gives us further information as to why we are not attaining the sense of wholeness we seek. Making a tape of one's own voice confirming one's needs and aspirations nurtures and strengthens the path of communication to one's deeper self.

Visualization is another means of bringing one's affirmation or desire to fruition. Regularly imagining oneself in the desired situation, and generating a feeling of worthiness from within, can be a powerful way of manifesting one's heart's desires. Gradually, with practice, old, limiting beliefs begin to recede and new, positive vibrations take their place. Practising visualization also enhances relaxation, helping us to move into a place of peace. It involves an inner exploration of our senses, whereby we imagine seeing, hearing, feeling, smelling, and touching objects or individuals that represent the object of our desires. A regular practice can be established, as follows. Sit in a comfortable chair, with your feet on the floor. Make sure you are comfortable and unlikely to be disturbed by noise or interruptions. Place a scarf or shawl around your shoulders to keep you warm. Close your eyes, and begin slow, mindful breathing. On the inhalation, allow the abdomen to expand, and feel the breath move into the chest. On the exhalation, feel all tension releasing from your neck, shoulders, arms and hands. As you continue the slow, rhythmic breathing, feel all tension leaving your torso, legs, and feet. Now imagine yourself in a meadow, high on a hillside. The long grass is dotted with wild flowers, and crimson poppies nod in the gentle breeze. Imagine yourself lying down in this meadow, feeling the sun warm your body. Taste the fragrant air as you breathe in, and feel your body relax even more as you exhale. You may visualize birds flying high in the sky above you, or imagine hearing the sound of insects chirping in the grass beside you. Engage as many of your senses as possible to make this image seem real. This private sanctuary can be used purely for relaxation, but also as a place where you can visualize the manifestation of your desires.

You may wish to tape-record a guided visualization for yourself, or to use one of the many pre-recorded ones available from bookstores. Created by well-known authors and speakers, these audio-cassettes deal with subjects such as addictions, eating disorders, loss of a loved one through separation or death, and manifesting what you want in life.

"Work in the invisible world at least as much as you do in the visible," advised the great Persian poet, Jalal-ud Din Rumi. His words are a reminder that, as we transport our minds through colour, meditation, chanting, music, and visualization, we are in the very rich world of the invisible.

In 1986, an extraordinary event occurred on this North American continent. John Randolph Price, the author of *The Angels Within Us,* was led through divine guidance to arrange a global mind link. He invited people around the planet to join in a worldwide meditation and prayer for peace. Each country and continent was synchronized to commence together. Based on computer analysis, millions of people were involved, and the numbers continue to grow for what is now an annual event. The timeframe for Western Canada is 4am on December 31 of each year. In the early years of this worldwide meditation, a friend and I would wrap ourselves in warm blankets and sit outside by the ponds at Thistledown to join in the meditation. Surrounded by trees, the soft darkness and, sometimes, stormy skies, we felt transported as we sat quietly for about an hour. Then we would move into the house for an early breakfast before the household was awake. For the rest of the day, before the New Year's Eve celebrations began, we felt connected and part of something larger than our daily lives—a very small part of a huge body caring for this planet of ours.

Price's book was the outcome of divine guidance given to him while he pursued his own healing path. This book is an exploration and explanation of the twenty-two angel archetypes, each describing an aspect of ourselves for our deeper understanding. Carl Jung described archetypes as the innate symbolic images that come from ancient stories, that are significant to individuals and cultures that help us to understand the human condition. A series of deep meditations and visions opened John Randolph Price's mind to the angelic realm and to learning how that realm is willing to connect with us on this plane. He describes his first meeting with the Angel of Creative Wisdom. When he asked the radiant being, "Do you have a name?" a soft, yet powerful, feminine voice said, "Some have called me Isis." The existence of angels has been recognized and taught since the establishment of spiritual brotherhoods and mystery schools thousands of years ago. The great classical art forms often depicted angels as chubby, winged cherubs floating above holy settings. John Randolph Price learned and wrote of other angels whose energies can reach into and affect individuals' lives—if those individuals are willing to receive them.

Each chapter in this insightful book ends with a meditation appropriate for seeking the qualities of each angelic archetype—a sort of update on Carl Jung's earlier work on the archetypes and their influences we carry within us. Price's examples of angelic conversations, meditations and exercises are for the purpose of uncovering our ego projections that block us from working with the angelic energy. I wanted to understand and access these energies.

I found the following angels particularly interesting and helpful at the latter stage of my healing journey: the Angel of Unconditional Love, which was about learning to love others as we have learned to love the self, with no strings attached; the Angel of Order and Harmony, which was about seeking a balance between head and heart, listening and speaking, stillness and action, while moving towards peace and serenity; and the angel of Loving Relationships, which was related to responsibility—the ability to respond to that which is needed by another, without undermining that individual's own responsibility.

But the angel I was most drawn to was the Angel of Discernment, which is the angel that the mystics of the East considered to be the Archetype of Karmic Deliverance. Karma is the Law of Cause and Effect—action and reaction—taught as part of 'natural science' in the ancient sacred academies. This angel is best called upon in moments of solitude to train the mind to be prudent and judicious, and to help you take action based on proper discernment.

The Angel of Discernment is also described as the Hermit, which I first saw depicted in a painting. It portrayed a monk-like figure, standing before a door illuminated by the light of a lantern he holds aloft. In his right hand, he carried a staff. The picture reminded me of the biblical instruction, "Knock and it shall be opened unto you." I was so drawn to this picture that I bought it and, for years, it hung on the wall beside my bedroom altar at Thistledown.

The Hermit is also featured in the tarot card deck, portrayed as an old man denoting prudence and circumspection.

On one occasion, when I needed clarity to solve a puzzling situation, I decided to call upon the Angel of Discernment for some perceptive guidance. I received an almost immediate response. I felt this presence, behind my right shoulder, and a hand enfolding mine. It happened so quickly, I felt I needed reassurance as to what I was doing, so I asked, "Will you tell me your name?" In a flash, without hesitation, came the name Adonis. According to Greek mythology, Adonis was a handsome youth. I returned to the Price material, and was happy to find that the Angel of Discernment (the Hermit) was indeed known as Adonis in some of the mystery schools. Through this presence, I received the understanding that, through the practice of heightened perception and discernment, we can begin to sense our real inner freedom. This, I believe, is what our soul stirrings lead us to do on this life's journey.

The Angel of Unconditional Love and Freedom relates to the unfolding of spiritual consciousness and initiation into a higher order of life. With this angel's help and, with hope, through the worldwide prayer connection, we may become conduits for bringing this understanding of inner freedom into the next century.

Another of John Randolph Price's books, *Angel Energy*, presents more information on this fascinating subject. Most of it is anecdotal material describing many of his readers' own experiences.

To be actively creative, we need to remove the blocks that prevent us from expressing our unique creative gifts. A delightful book written for the purpose of reminding us how to rediscover the art of expressing ourselves creatively is Julia Cameron's *The Artist's Way: a Spiritual Path to Higher Creativity.* Cameron leads us through a comprehensive twelve-week program of recovery from a variety of blocks that could be impeding our very personal and unique expressions. This book links creativity to personal empowerment through learnable skills, effective exercises, and activities that spur the imagination to capture new ideas. It can be a gift to you from you, as my copy was for me.

The basic tools in this program are the Morning Pages and the Artist's Date. The Morning Pages are a regular morning ritual involving three pages of longhand writing that is strictly stream of consciousness. These daily meanderings on paper are the very first activity of the day and contain whatever you want to talk about to yourself. Nobody is allowed to read your Morning Pages, and even the writer is encouraged not to read them for eight weeks. The Morning Pages requires a thick notebook, an assortment of pens, stickers and stars to decorate the cover. This book will become the repository of your true feelings. My past journal writings always had the sense of a third party looking over my shoulder. This feeling quickly dissipates as the exercises invite the child, the young man or woman, the mature self, the crone, and the sage to come and share their wisdom with us. There is nothing that cannot be told, and nothing that will be divulged without the permission of that aspect of our being.

An Artist's Date is a regular date you make with yourself for nurturing creative consciousness, and you take no one on this date but your inner artist—also known as your creative child. This can be the beginning of some very interesting 'dates' you take yourself on over the course of twelve weeks. Through this process, I found a new sense of respect and desire in expressing my ways of being creative. One doesn't have to be an artist in the literal or accepted sense. In whatever way we creatively express ourselves, that is our art!

I still do my Morning Pages. Initially, they were speckled with '*why me?*' and '*I can't*' but I have moved on to better things now. The Morning Pages make me feel good; they sometimes surprise me, and they often make me laugh at myself. In 1996, Julia Cameron came to Vancouver to give a workshop (or 'playshop,' as she liked to call it), to introduce her latest book, *Vein of Gold—Journey to your Creative Heart*. She was accompanied by Tim Wheater, a musician who, through illness, had lost the use of the muscles around his lips and could no longer play the music he composed for his flute. After he had passed through the 'Valley of Despair,' he began training his voice to create a flute-like sound that allowed him to continue composing. Eventually, his lips healed, and he can now play and make music that is a blend of vocal, instrumental, aboriginal and toning sounds that were electrifying to those of us in the gathering. A further creative miracle happened when Julia Cameron went to Tim for voice lessons to see if she, too, could recover from her childhood block of being the 'groaner' in a family of prominent musicians. She sang for us some of the amazing music she channelled during the course of her time with Tim Wheater, some of which has now been expanded into a fully-fledged musical. This wonderful exchange was an inspiring example of how opening to our creativity can unlock and open doors within ourselves that we would never dream we had. As we witnessed these two teachers who walked their talk in a way I had never experienced before, they gave us proof that we all had the capacity to do the same.

I give myself the first two hours of the day, and I cherish this time. I now know that this illness has given me the opportunity to learn wonderful healing lessons that I could not have learned otherwise. Instead of helping others to heal, I was forced to make myself the focus of my healing work. I was given the opportunity and the motivation to look more deeply inside myself for answers to questions I might otherwise never have asked.

I would like to share the following insightful passage from Julia Cameron's book, *The Artist's Way*:

> *Above all, God is the source. No human power can deflect our good or create it. We are all conduits for a higher self that would work through us. We are all equally connected to a spiritual source. We do not always know which among us will teach us best. We are all meant to cherish and serve one another. The Artist's Way is tribal. The spirit of service yields us our dharma—that right path we dream of following in our best and most fulfilled moments of faith.*

Chapter 11 / Your Healing Journey

Our world is what we think it is.
If we can change our thoughts,
we can change our world.
—H. M. Tomlinson

Chronic illness is one of the ways your body, mind and spirit cry out in a desperate, last-ditch attempt to get your attention. They are trying to tell you that your soul yearns for a deeper knowledge of who you are, and that, deep inside, you have all the resources to help and heal yourself. And this healing is rarely just of the illness at hand; it pertains to deeply buried issues that require dedicated excavation, and that inevitably lead to greater personal knowledge and fulfilment.

My healing story spans over seven years, but I do believe that, in even seven weeks, you can make many small changes to alleviate some of your pain and discomfort.

You are probably wondering where you will find the time in a busy schedule to fit it all in. Time is what our lives are made of, and both time and life are ultimately ours to use as we choose. If we have become crippled by disease, our only choice is to give time to our healing process.

Begin by nurturing yourself as well as, if not better than, you nurture those around you. If possible, make a private space somewhere in your living quarters for a comfortable chair, books, note pad and pens, and a cozy blanket for napping. Take time to go into a receptive, meditative state, and ask yourself if you have any information to help you understand when this condition could have started. Remembering childhood scenes, youthful dreams and adult experiences is important. This will reveal not only the pain and discomfort that cause illness, but will also reconnect you with the memories of the sheer, uncomplicated joy of childhood that is so valuable on your healing journey. Let your inner being feel your love and sincere desire to know what you need to know to help you back to wholeness. Be gentle with yourself. Speak to yourself using a name that engenders feelings of love, and remember that every one of us has always done the very best we could with the information and awareness available to us at the time. You are the most important person in your life right now, and if your mind says, "I can't be," let your heart say, "I would like it to be so."

As Ernest Homes, Founder of the Church of Religious Science, says, "We all have the ability to transcend previous experiences and rise triumphant above them, but we shall never triumph over them while we persist in going through the old mental reactions."

By rising one hour earlier (and retiring one hour earlier), you can begin the shift to finding the time you need. Make enquiries of other family members if there is a history of food allergies you are not aware of. Perhaps you have sensed there are changes you would like to make in the way you perceive yourself dealing with osteoarthritis. Most changes do require help from others, but we need to be armed with the information to make those choices that will bring us back to good health.

Check your medical coverage. Fees for some alternative therapies are partially covered by your medical plan. If you feel your doctor is receptive, discuss your plans to become an active participant in your healing process. Ask him or her to refer you to a massage therapist. While joints are inflamed, they are not to be rubbed, but gentle stroking of neck and back will allow you to relax. Later, full-body massages will be most beneficial.

A reflexology treatment is a very relaxing, non-threatening way to experience hands-on manipulation of your body. As the feet tell their own story, the reflexologist will help you understand and monitor what is happening physically.

Enquire about chiropractors who practise kinesiology, or muscle testing, as a way of asking your body for information before treatment begins. People with arthritis tend to tense themselves so as not to feel pain, and this puts the body out of alignment, placing undue strain on muscles and ligaments. Long-standing pain can be relieved and often eliminated with these approaches.

Ask other healthcare practitioners about selecting a competent naturopathic physician, and look in your local papers for advertisements of new naturopathic clinics starting in your area. It is important to ask if he or she offers Vega Testing for determining your food plan. Also ask if homeopathic remedies and advice on a vitamin supplement program are available. Remember that it is a kindness to yourself to ask questions if you do not feel clear about anything. This is your part in your healing program.

Healthfood stores are wonderful sources of information. Usually the staff members are well informed and have a supply of free health journals and magazines that publish up-to-date information from reliable sources.

Start your day with a walk, no matter how short or slow. Just get out and breathe! Before attending any exercise class, make the instructor aware of any difficulties you are having. Tai Chi is a gentle way to start loosening up neck, shoulders, hips, knees and ankles. The exercises are slow and fluid, giving you a sense of being unhurried. A swimming pool where Aquafit classes are taught can be most beneficial. The buoyancy of the water takes the weight off sore limbs while exercising. Public swimming pools often have a hot tub to soothe tired muscles and joints.

New and second-hand bookstores and libraries are an Ali Baba's cave of information, helping you to make informed choices. The Internet is another invaluable source of up-to-date information about holistic healing. Bookstores and healthfood stores often advertise workshops on holistic healing practices, usually including an introductory evening with only a nominal charge. Go with a friend and enjoy exploring together.

Vegetarian cooking classes may also provide helpful tips for your new regimen. Some classes include cooking with the newly discovered grains and beans, and their appropriate seasonings, to make delicious healthy meals. If you find you are allergic to dairy products, the good news is that soy milks now on the market are a far cry from the early gritty ones, that bore little resemblance to real milk.

An essential part of your healing regimen is your evening bath. You will need the following items for maximum benefit:

- 1 cup each of bath-quality Epson salts and baking soda.
- Edible almond oil (available in your healthfood store cooler). It is not as expensive as massage oil.
- A long-handled brush with soft bristles, or skin exfoliating gloves, to dry-brush your body.

Allow yourself forty-five minutes of undisturbed time. Add the Epsom salts and baking soda under running water to dissolve them, together with one tablespoon of almond oil and a dash of liquid bath soap. Fill up the rest of the bath with comfortably warm-to-hot water, adding a few drops of lavender/geranium aromatherapy oil for body relaxation.

Before getting into the bath, begin dry-brushing, as described in Chapter 4. Our skin is the largest organ of the body, and brushing it loosens dead skin, allowing the pores to breathe and the internal toxins to be released. Your circulation will be enhanced and your skin will glow.

Step into the bath, immersing yourself from neck to toe. Wring out a washcloth and place it over your face for a few minutes. Feel your facial muscles softening and letting go. Consciously let go of tension in every part of your body until you feel completely relaxed. It helps to sigh loudly as you do this.

After twenty minutes of soaking, release the bath water and kneel or stand in the bottom of the tub. Rinse off with either a hand spray or a jug of tepid water. Step out of the tub and enfold yourself in a warm towel. Pat yourself dry.

Warm two or three tablespoons of almond oil between your palms and rub on your elbows, knees and feet to soften the skin. Hop into bed feeling totally relaxed and nurtured.

You have started your own healing journey.

Epilogue

In the summer of 1995, my friend Louise asked me to go ballooning with her on her sixtieth birthday. I was delighted. We met at 6am on a Saturday morning, on the far side of the airfield, where a huge, striped, half-filled balloon lay. It was being brought to life by blasts of heat, needed to carry us aloft. The small basket attached to the guy wires looked rather small to carry nine of us. When all was made ready, the pilot called, "Right-oh, hop aboard," and we lined up. My foot found the mounting hole in the side of the basket, my hands reached up to grasp the basket top, and I hoisted up, flinging my other leg over the side and hopping in. I took my place with the other seven passengers lined around the basket ready for take off.

The view from above was breathtakingly beautiful. The only sound was from the gas flame that kept us aloft and the gentle wind that floated us upward. As I watched the farms and fields grow smaller, and the model villages far below, I felt as elated as I had been on my first childhood donkey ride. But there was an added sense of delight. I had actually 'hopped aboard.' I pulled my cap down tighter on my head and savoured the sense of freedom up there in the sky and the feeling of having come such a long way from the day I dropped the hot teapot on my kitchen floor.

On our descent, the pilot negotiated a small copse of alder trees and a large green stagnant pond. Then we were scudding down into long grass, gradually coming to a stop. We climbed out of the basket and wandered about in the tall grasses as the ground crew appeared in the field to empty and pack the magnificent balloon onto a jeep. We returned to the airfield to a gazebo set to one side where drinks of champagne and orange juice awaited us in tall cold glasses. As we toasted one another, the pilot handed each one of us his signed statement from the Fantasy Balloon Charters. It declared that, on this day, we had been transported by said balloon. The sheet also carried the ballooner's poem.

The winds have welcomed you with softness
The sun has blessed you with warm hands
You have flown so high and so well
that God has joined you in laughter
And has set you gently back again
into the loving arms of Mother Earth.

This memento of that day hangs on the wall above my desk. It is an 'open sesame' for me to embrace the challenges and joy that my vibrant good health draws toward me.

I wish you peace and joy on your healing journey.

Blessings,
Audrey Buchanan, 2000

Selected References & Further Reading

Anatomy of an Illness, Norman Cousins, MD. Published by Bantam Books, 10 East 53rd St, New York, NY, USA.

Ancient Wisdom Revealed—the Soul Journey Discourses, Craig Russel. Published by So Be It Productions, 7073 Adera St, Vancouver, BC, V6P 5CS.

The Angels within Us, John Randolph Price; *Angel Energy,* John Randolph Price. Published by Ballantine Books Div. of Random House Inc., New York, NY, USA.

The Aquarian Conspiracy, Personal and Social Transformation, Marilyn Ferguson. Published by J.P. Tarcher Inc., 911 Sunset Blvd, Los Angeles, CA 90069, USA.

The Arthritis Handbook: the Complete Guide to Living a Healthy, Productive Life with Arthritis, Theodore W. Rooney, D.O. & Patty Ryan Rooney. Published by Random House of Canada Limited, Toronto, Ontario, Canada, 1989.

Arthritis—the Allergy Connection, Dr John Mansfield. Published by Thorsons Harper Collins, 77-85 Fulham Palace Rd, London W8 W6 8JB.

The Artist's Way, Julia Cameron. Published by Putnam Publishing Group, 200 Madison Ave, New York, NY, USA.

Awareness through Movement, Moshe Feldenkrais. Published by Harper & Row, 10 East 53rd St, New York, NY, 10022, USA.

The Ayurvedic Cookbook: a Personalized Guide to Good Nutrition and Health, Amadea Morningstar with Urmila Desai. Published by Lotus Light, PO Box 2, Wilmot, WI 53192, USA. 1990.

Ayurveda—the Science of Self-Healing, Dr Vasant Lad. Published by Lotus Press, PO Box 6265 Santa Fe, New Mexico, USA.

Behavioural Kinesiology, John Diamond, MD. Published by Harper & Row Inc., 10 East 53rd St, New York, NY 10022, USA.

Brain Gym Handbook, Paul Dennison, PhD, and Gail Dennison. Published by Edu-Kinesthetics Inc., Ventura, California.

Care of the Soul, Thomas Moore. Published by Harper Collins Inc., 10 E. 53rd St, New York, NY 10022, USA.

The Celestine Prophecy, James Redfield. Published by Time Warner Books Inc., New York, NY 10020, USA.

Complete Book of Essential Oils, Valerie Ann Worwood, published by New World Library, Novatu, California, USA.

The Complete Illustrated Holistic Herbal, David Hoffman. Published by The Findhorn Press, Findhorn, Moray, Scotland, UK.

Conversations with God, Books I and II, Neale Donald Walsch. Published by Hampton Roads Publishing Inc., 134 Burgess Lane, Charlottesville, VA 22902, USA.

A Course in Miracles, Foundation for Inner Peace, PO Box 635, Tiburon, California 94920, USA.

Creative Thought: the Magazine of Daily Inspirations, PO Box 2152, Spokane, Washington, USA.

Dashan: in the Company of Saints, SYDA Foundation, PO Box 600, South Falsbury, NY 12779, USA.

The Edgar Cayce Handbook for Health through Drugless Therapy, published by Dr Harold J. Reilly and Ruth Hagy Brod.

The Edgar Cayce Remedies, William McGary, MD. Published by Bantam Books, Canada

Embrace Tiger Return to Mountain, Al Huang. Published by Celestial Arts Publishing, PO Box 7327, Berkeley, California 94707, USA.

Emerson's Essays, Ralph Waldo Emerson. Published by Thomas Y. Crowell Co., New York, NY, USA.

Energy Medicine: Pacific Flower and Sea Essences, Sabina Pettitt, Pacific Essences, 403 Kingston St, Victoria, BC, Canada.

Fit for Life, Harvey and Marilyn Diamond. Published by Warner Books, 1271 Avenue of Americas, New York, NY 10020, USA.

Flower Essences, Machaelle Wright. Published by Perelendra Ltd, PO Box 36003, Warrenton, VA 94920, USA.

Flower Essence Services, PO Box 1769, Nevada City, CA 95959, USA.

Fragrant Mind, Valerie Ann Worwood. Published by New World Library, Novatu, California, USA.

Freedom from Allergy Cookbook, Ron Greenberg, MD, and Angela Nori. Published by Blue Poppy Press, 212-2678 West Broadway, Vancouver, BC, V6K 2G3, Canada.

Gem Elixirs & Vibrational Healing, Guradas through Kevin Ryerson. Published by Cassandra Press, Boulder 80306, USA.

Goodbye to Guilt, Gerald Jampolsky, MD. Published by Bantam Books Inc., 666 Fifth Ave, New York, NY 10103, USA.

Handbook of the Bach Flower Remedies, Phillip M. Chancellor. The C. W. Daniel Co. Ltd, 60 Muswell Road, London, N10, UK.

A Harp Full of Stars, Joel Andrew. Published by Golden Harp Press, PO Box 335, Ben Lomond, CA 95004, USA. (Cassettes and CDs available.)

Healing for the Age of Enlightenment, Stanley Burroughs. PO Box 260, Kailua, HI 96734, USA.

Healing into life and Death, Stephen Levine. Published by Doubleday, 1540 Broadway, New York, NY 10036, USA.

Health through God's Pharmacy, Maria Trebe. Wilhelm Ennsthaler, Steyr, Austria.

Healthy...Naturally, by Michele Boisvert (order from Alive, PO Box 80055, Burnaby, BC, V5H 3X1, Canada).

The Herb Book, John Lust ND, DBM. Published by Benedict Lust Publications, 490 East St, Sini Valley, CA 93065, USA.

Hildegard of Bingen's Medicine, Dr Wighard Strehlow and Gottfried Strehlow. Published by Bear Co., PO Drawer 2860, Santa Fe, New Mexico 87504, USA.

Holy Man, Susan Trott. Published by Rivermead Books, 200 Madison Avenue, New York, NY 10016, USA.

The Homeopathic Home Care Kit: a User's Guide, Neil Tessler, ND. Published by Homeomed Associates, Fernadale, WA, 98248, USA.

How to Get Well, Paavo Airola, PhD ND. Published by Health Plus Publishers, PO Box 22001, Phoenix, AS, USA.

In Tune with the Infinite, Ralph Waldo Trine. Published by G. Bell and Sons, London, England, UK.

Inner Cleansing: How to Free Yourself from Joint-Muscle-Artery-Circulation Sludge, Carlson Wade. Published by Parker Publishing Co. Inc., West Nyack, NY, USA, 1993.

Joy of Cooking, Irma S. Rambauer and Marion Rambauer Becker. Published by New American Library Inc., 1301 Avenue of the Americas, New York, NY 10019, USA.

Know Your Nutrition, Linda Clark, MA. Published by Keats Publishing Inc., CT, USA.

Let's Get Well, Adelle Davis. Published by Harcourt, Brace and World Inc., New York, NY, USA.

Listening to the Body, Robert Masters, PhD & Jean Houston PhD,

Published by Dell Publishing Co. Inc., Daag Hammerskjold Plaza, New York, NY 10017, USA.

Love is Letting Go of Fear, Gerald Jampolsky, MD. Published by Bantam Books, Celestial Arts, 231 Adrian Road Millbrae, CA 9403, USA.

The McDougall Program: Twelve Days to Dynamic Health, John A. McDougall, MD. Published by Penguin Books Canada Ltd, Markham, Ontario, Canada, 1991.

MAP—the Co-creative White Brotherhood Medical Assistance Program, Machaelle Small Wright. Published by Perelandra Ltd, PO Box 3603, Warrenton, VA 20188, USA.

The Medical Discoveries of Edward Bach Physician, Nora Weeks. Published by C. W. Daniel and Co. Ltd, 60 Muswell Road, London N10, UK.

The Metamorphic Technique: Principles and Practice, Gaston Saint-Pierre and Debbie Boater. Published by Element Books Ltd, The Old Brewery, Tisbury, Wiltshire, UK.

The Nature and Health Journal, Neville Drury, Sydney, Australia.

New Bach Flower Body Maps—Treatment by Topical Application, Dietmar Kramer. Published by Healing Arts Press, Rochester, Vermont, US.

Passion for Life, John James & Muriel James. Published by Penguin Books USA Inc., 375 Hudson St, New York, NY 10014, USA.

The Path to Love, Deepak Chopra, MD. Published by Harmony Books, 201 East 50th St, New York, NY 10022, USA.

Perelandra Centre for Nature Research, PO Box 3603, Warrenton, VA 22186, USA.

Perfect Health: the Complete Mind-Body Guide, Deepak Chopra, MD. Published by Harmony books, 201 East 50th St New York, NY 10022, USA.

The Possible Human, Jean Houston. Published by J.P. Archer Inc., 9110 Sunset Blvd, Los Angeles, CA 90069, USA.

The Pritikin Program, Nathan Pritikin with Patrick M. McGrady Jr. Published by Grosset & Dunlap, New York, USA.

Relaxercize, based on *The Easy New Way to Health and Fitn*ess, Dr Moshe Feldenkrais, Bersin, Bersin and Reese, Published by Harper's San Francisco, CA, USA.

Self-Discovery Directory, published by *Shared Vision Magazine*, 203-873 Beatty St, Vancouver, BC, V6B 2M6, Canada.

Seven Herbs: Plants as Teachers, Mathew Wood. Published by North Atlantic Books, Berkeley, CA, USA.

Seven Laws for Success, Deepak Chopra, MD. Published by Harmony Books, 201 East 50th St, New York, NY 10022, USA.

Shiatsu, Wataru Ohashi. Published by Clarke, Irwin and Co. Ltd, Vancouver, BC, Canada.

Stand Tall, Morris Notelovitz, MD, & Marsha Ware. Published by Bantam Books, 666 Fifth Avenue, New York, NY 10103, USA.

Stories the Feet Can Tell, Eunice D. Ingram. Published by Ingram Publishers, PO Box 8412, Rochester, New York 14618, USA.

The Tassajara Recipe Book, Edward Espe Brown. Published by Shambala Publications, 300 Massachusetts Ave, Boston, MASS 02115, USA.

Teach Only Love, the Principles of Attitudinal Healing, G. Jampolsky, MD. Published by Bantam Books Inc., 66 Fifth Avenue, New York, NY 10103, USA.

There is a Cure for Arthritis, Paavo O. Airola, ND. Published by Health Plus Publishers, Phoenix, AZ, USA.

Tissue Cleansing through Bowel Management, Bernard Jensen, DC.

Toxemia, John H. Tilden, MD. Published by American Society, Natural Hygiene Society Inc., Bridgeport, Connecticut 06604, USA.

The Twelve Healers, Edward Bach. Published by The CW Daniel Co. Ltd, London, UK.

Vegan Delights, Jeanne Marie Martin. Published by Harbour Publishing, Madiera Park, BC, Canada.

The Vein of Gold—a Journey to your Creative Heart. Published by Putnam Publishing Group, 200 Madison Ave, New York, NY, USA.

Vibrational Medicine, New Choices for Healing Ourselves, Richard Gerber, MD. Published by Bear & Co., Santa Fe, New Mexico, USA.

148

The Way to Vibrant Health, Alexander Lowen MD, & LeslieLowen. Published by Harper Colophon Books, 10 East 53rd. St, New York, NY 10022, USA.

You Can Heal Your Life, Louise Hay. Published by Hay House, 3029 Wilshire Blvd, Santa Monica, CA 90404, USA.

About the Author

Audrey G. Buchanan was born in Surrey, England, and came to Canada in 1952. In the early 60s, she became interested in natural holistic living and alternative healing methods. Through training and extensive research, she quickly developed an in-depth knowledge of the principles of body/mind healing and became a holistic practitioner in 1978. A chartered herbalist (certified by the Dominion Herbal College of BC), and a counsellor in the progressive Sentinel High School Alternative Program of West Vancouver, BC, she also trained at the Holistic Health Institute of Santa Cruz, in California, and was a member of the Hatha Yoga Teachers Association of BC.

Her practice in West Vancouver, and on the Sunshine Coast, BC, included holistic Swedish-Esalen massage, bodywork, diet and exercise programs, herbal, Flower Remedies, and workshops.

At 73, she continues to lead an active, healthy life on the Sunshine Coast, BC, in retirement with her husband Ross. She loves to travel, paint, cook and work in their garden.